BRITISH ARMY AMBULANCE TRAINS

BRIAN ROBERTSON

AMBERLEY

About the Author

Colonel (retd) Brian Robertson was born in North London and educated at Highgate School. He attended the Royal Free Hospital School of Medicine, in London, and qualified as a doctor in 1972. His military service started in the Territorial Army in 1965 in 167 (City of London) Field Ambulance RAMC/TA. He was appointed to a Medical Cadetship in 1970 and following a short service Regular Commission in the Royal Army Medical Corps he transferred to the Army Medical Services TA. He spent fifteen years training and operating ambulance trains within the British Army of the Rhine during the latter years of the Cold War. Between 1985 and 1994 he held the appointment of Squadron Commander of the Ambulance Train Squadron RAMC(V) in the rank of Lieutenant Colonel. With the end of the Cold War all British Army Ambulance Train capability was disbanded. He was subsequently promoted and appointed to command 306 Field Hospital (V) between 1995 and 1999 and eventually retired from the Army in December 2007.

Front cover, top: One of two ambulance trains deployed on Exercise FLYING SCOT 93 at Hohne; *bottom*: A DB Class 216 locomotive waiting to depart with an ambulance train at Sennelager in 1993. *Back cover*: The Princess Christian Hospital Train before deployment. (British Red Cross Museum and Archives)

First published 2025

Amberley Publishing
The Hill, Stroud
Gloucestershire, GL5 4EP

www.amberley-books.com

British Library Cataloguing in Publication Data.

A catalogue record for this book is available from the British Library.

ISBN 978 1 3981 2343 4 (print)
ISBN 978 1 3981 2344 1 (ebook)

Origination by Amberley Publishing.
Printed in the UK.

Appointed GPSR EU Representative: Easy Access System Europe Oü, 16879218
Address: Mustamäe tee 50, 10621, Tallinn, Estonia
Contact Details: gpsr.requests@easproject.com, +358 40 500 3575

Acronyms and Abbreviations

AEF	American Expeditionary Force
AF	Army Form
AMS	Army Medical Services
APO	Army Post Office
BAOR	British Army of the Rhine
BDA	*Béchôt-Déspres-Amelines*
BEF	British Expeditionary Force
BR	British Railways
C&W	Carriage and Wagon
CAT	Continental ambulance train
CCS	Casualty Clearing Station
CET	Casualty evacuation train
Comm Z	Communication Zone
DB	*Deutsches Bahn*
DR	*Deutsches Reichsbahn*
Etat	*Chemin de Fer de l'État*
FAU	Friends' Ambulance Unit
FCZ	Forward Combat Zone
FO	First Open
FSC	Forward Surgical Complex
ft	Feet
GCR	Great Central Railway
GER	Great Eastern Railway
GWR	Great Western Railway
HAT	Home ambulance train
HMHS	His Majesty's hospital ship
hp	Horsepower
HQ	Headquarters
HS	Hospital ship
IEF	Indian Expeditionary Force
IMS	Indian Medical Services
ins	Inches
JTP	Joint Theatre Plan
KCB	Knight Commander of the Order of the Bath

km	Kilometre
LBSCR	London, Brighton & South Coast Railway
LMS	London, Midland & Scottish Railway
LNWR	London & North Western Railway
LoC	Line of Communications
L/Sgt	Lance Sergeant
LST	Landing Ship Tank
LSWR	London & South Western Railway
Lt Col	Lieutenant Colonel
LYR	Lancashire and Yorkshire Railway
m	Metre
MBE	Member of the Order of the British Empire
MEDEVAC	Emergency evacuation of sick and wounded
MEDLOC	Mediterranean Line of Communication
MO	Medical Officer
MoD	Ministry of Defence
MoH	Ministry of Health
MR	Midland Railway
MSC	Medical Staff Corps
MSF	*Médecins Sans Frontières*
NATO	North Atlantic Treaty Organisation
NCO	Non-commissioned officer
NER	North Eastern Railway
NO	Nursing officer
Nord	*Chemin de Fer du Nord*
OAT	Overseas ambulance train
OR	Other rank
ORBAT	Order of battle
PLM	*Chemin de Fer de Paris à Lyon et à la Méditerrannée*
PoW	Prisoner of war
QAIMNS	Queen Alexandra's Imperial Military Nursing Service
QARANC	Queen Alexandra's Royal Army Nursing Corps
QARNNS	Queen Alexandra's Royal Naval Nursing Service
RAF	Royal Air Force
RAMC	Royal Army Medical Corps
RCC	Railway Construction Company
RCT	Royal Corps of Transport
RCZ	Rear Combat Zone
RE	Royal Engineers
REME	Royal Electrical and Mechanical Engineers
Retd	Retired
RLC	Royal Logistic Corps
RMS	Royal Mail Ship
RN	Royal Navy

ROD	Railway Operating Division
Ro-Ro	Roll-on, roll-off
RPC	Royal Pioneer Corps
SECR	South East & Chatham Railway
SJAB	St John Ambulance Brigade
SMOM	Sovereign Military Order of Malta
SNCF	*Société Nationale des chemins de fer Français*
SNCO	Senior non-commissioned officer
SR	Southern Railway
SS	Steamship
STUFT	Ships taken up from trade
TA	Territorial Army
TGV	*Train à grande vitesse*
TTW	Transition to war
VAD	Voluntary Aid Detachment
WD	War Department
WHO	World Health Organisation
UK	United Kingdom
UN	United Nations
US	United States
USA	United States of America
USATC	United States Army Transportation Corps

Preface

During almost every military campaign since the invention of railways, ambulance and hospital trains have made a major contribution. They have been used in one form or another wherever railways have existed. However, they rarely rate more than a few lines in campaign histories, yet they have a long and distinguished past along with a story that needs to be told.

The aim of this work is to offer a chronological history of ambulance train operating by, on behalf of, or connected to the British Military. This work will follow the evolution of moving sick and wounded since the earliest days of rail in the Crimean War, through the South African War and both world wars up to the end of the Cold War.

In 1905 the Spanish-American philosopher George Santayana is credited with the quote 'Those who cannot remember the past are condemned to repeat it.' This is of major importance as so often the lessons from the past are not heeded and the same actions and implied mistakes are repeated by a future generation. What is commonly referred to as the loss of corporate memory has been applied to military matters in the following terms: '…there is historical evidence of the loss of collective knowledge between wars'.[1]

This has been the case when one looks at the history of ambulance trains. Britain disbanded its entire ambulance train capability after the First World War. The capability that was reinvented was drastically reduced again after the Second World War and then completely disbanded after the Cold War. At the time of writing the need for ambulance trains in Europe is being discussed once again as a consequence of the war in Ukraine and the risk of a wider European conflict.

This work has gathered material from a wide range of sources, although it is somewhat difficult to know the primary source. Other authors have noted how incorrect facts are sometimes perpetuated from publication to publication. As has been mentioned, some campaign histories simply carry references to casualties being moved by rail with no detail as to the organisation, provisioning, conversion, staffing or operating of the trains in question. This work will try to build on those sketchy references to ensure that ambulance trains and those who converted them along with the staff who operated them are not forgotten.

I have been fortunate and privileged to have been given some personal testimony from veterans who served on ambulance trains during both the Second World War and the Korean War. Where included their memories add a very human element to this history. I also have an interest in the postal history of ambulance trains and the humble postcard, which had its heyday during the First World War, can sometimes reveal interesting facts about ambulance train operating.

Many people have given freely of their time and expertise to help with my research and have thus contributed to this finished work. I am very grateful to the following: Sarah-Jane Anscomb, Roger Aston, Rob Bayliff, Roger Farnworth, Charles Freil, Garry George, Clem Maginniss, Chen Melling, George Moon, Tim Pettis, Julian Rainbow, Walter Rothschild and Robin Thorne.

Reference will be made to a very detailed Second World War primary source of information that Graham and Anne Hudson have generously allowed me to utilise and quote in detail. The late Lt Col (retd) Leonard Hudson MBE had a career in the railway industry and was seconded from the Southern Railway to the Movements Directorate of the War Office to support the war effort. In 1992 Leonard Hudson gave me some of his personal records of the work with ambulance trains that he wrote in 1946, and they give a detailed insight into the planning for ambulance train operating during the Second World War. I must record my gratitude to his family for allowing me to ensure his historic records are not lost, and the contribution he made not forgotten.

I should also like to record my gratitude to the late John Poyntz whose friendship and encyclopaedic knowledge about railways in general and military railways in particular was always a constant source of encouragement. It is a great regret that he has not been able to critique my final draft.

Every attempt has been made to seek permission for copyright material used in this work. However, if copyright material has been used inadvertently, without permission or acknowledgement, apologies are offered and necessary corrections will be made at the first opportunity. The author and publisher would like to thank the following institutions and organisations, along with their representatives, for permission to use copyright material: Malcolm Boyns, Archivist, Bristol Archives; Stephen Noble, Archivist, British Red Cross Museum and Archives; Mark Trasler, Haslar Heritage Group; Andrew Webb, Licensing Executive, Imperial War Museum; Jason Semmens, Director, Museum of Military Medicine; Alison Kay, Senior Curator of Archives and the Staff of the Picture Library, National Railway Museum and David Harman of the Transport Ticket Society.

Thanks are also due to Sally Finlayson for the generation of the mapping and other artwork used in this work. Also, to Anne Willmott for considerable assistance cataloguing my entire ambulance train archive over many years, along with the repeated proofreading undertaken throughout the gestation of this work.

Thanks must also go to my daughters and their spouses, Katherine and Rudi, and Alison and Rob, for their constant support and encouragement with this and other projects and for listening with patience to my constant passion for 'all things ambulance trains'.

Finally, it must be stated that all errors and omissions are mine alone.

Brian Robertson
Ash, Surrey

Contents

1

Early Days of the Use of Railways

It is often quoted that Great Britain gave the world railways and it is certainly true that the British inventor Richard Trevithick (1771–1833) developed the high-pressure steam engine and, in 1804, built the first working steam locomotive that ran on wrought-iron rails.

The earliest recorded use of railways to move sick and wounded during warfare was in 1855 during the Crimean War (1853–56) when they were carried lying on straw in the open wagons that had been used to build a railway inland from Balaklava. The Grand Crimean Military Railway, as it came to be known, was built in 1855 by British engineering contractors Peto, Brassey and Betts.[1] Some 7 miles of track were laid with the purpose of improving the supply of ammunition and other stores to the British forces engaged in the siege of Sebastopol who were based on a plateau between Balaklava and Sebastopol. A new Land Transport Corps had been formed on 24 January 1855 to undertake what would now be called the logistics for an army in the field. This Land Transport Corps subsequently took over operating the railway from the contractors. Five steam locomotives from various British companies were shipped out to the Crimea and there were also three stationary winding engines that were used on the steepest part of the route.

On 2 April 1855 four wagons containing sick and wounded ran from the British Headquarters down to the port at Balaklava apparently in less than half an hour, significantly quicker than the previous dependence on horse and mule litters.[2] The first chapter in the history of the use of rail to transport sick and wounded in warfare had been written.

Despite having led the world in the development of railways, Great Britain did not lead the way in harnessing the potential of rail for casualty transportation. Trains were subsequently used in several wars including the American Civil War (1861–65), which was to become the first major conflict in which railways were to play an important role as their capability for moving troops, supplies and wounded was realised. Rolling stock that was specially converted was first introduced by the Union Forces in 1862 and these coaches carried twenty-four stretchers slung on heavy rubber bands. Hospital trains, as they were called by both armies, ran in all areas of the American Civil War and just one example of their use was in 1863 after the Battle of Gettysburg when 15,425 wounded were moved by rail between 7 and 22 July to hospitals in Baltimore, Harrisburg and New York.[3]

Great Britain took one small step in 1869 when the War Department requested the London & South Western Railway (LSWR) provide a means of conveying lying patients.[4] The LSWR had come into being in 1838 and existed until its amalgamation with other lines to form the Southern Railway in 1922. In 1870 the Metropolitan Carriage Works in Birmingham converted an ex-postal six-wheeled van to a design by Surgeon-General Sir Thomas Longmore.[5] Commonly referred to as the 'Admiralty' coach, this single coach could carry eight lying patients and was used to transfer patients from Portsmouth and Southampton Docks to Netley Station on the LSWR in order for them to reach the Royal Victoria Hospital. A second coach was converted between 1885 and 1886, but very little detail has survived.

In Europe, although rail had been used in a primitive way in several minor wars there were three major events that were to shape the development of the use of rail for casualty transportation for many years to come. These were the Franco-Prussian War of 1870–71 and somewhat surprisingly the 1873 Vienna World's Fair followed by the 1876 International Exhibition and Congress of Public Health and Safety that was held in Brussels.

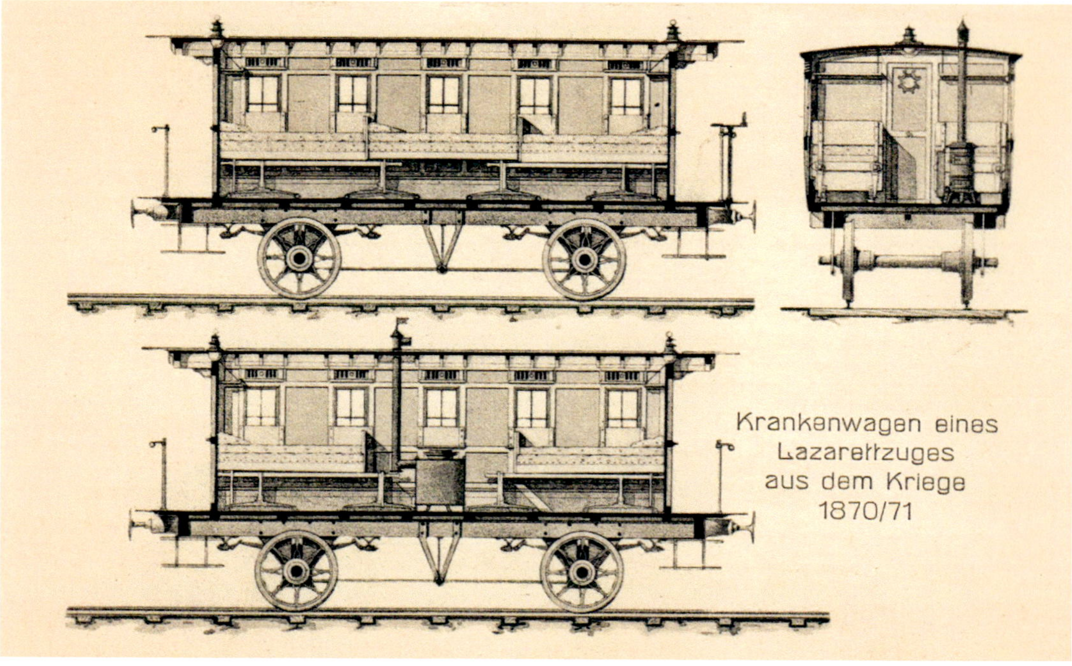

A four-wheeled coach as used within a hospital train operated during the Franco-Prussian War of 1870–71.

The Franco-Prussian War was a conflict between the Second French Empire and the North German Confederation led by the Kingdom of Prussia. The outcome was a German victory that led to the unification of German States with the creation of the German Empire along with the German annexation of Alsace-Lorraine from France. What is important in the context of this work is that it was during the Franco-Prussian War that purpose-designed hospital trains were created and operated by the Prussian Army. Twenty-one trains were utilised and over 89,000 patients were carried by rail during the conflict.[6]

Following the Franco-Prussian War there was increased development of hospital train capabilities. This was given a significant boost by the Vienna World's Fair that was held between May and November 1873 and welcomed over 7 million visitors. Several international exhibitors presented their ideas specifically in relation to hospital and ambulance trains.

The International Exhibition and Congress of Public Health and Safety followed in Brussels, Belgium, in 1876 and the subject of ambulance rail transport continued to be featured. The Exhibition and Congress was divided into ten classes of which the fourth was devoted to the provision of 'aid to belligerents in time of war

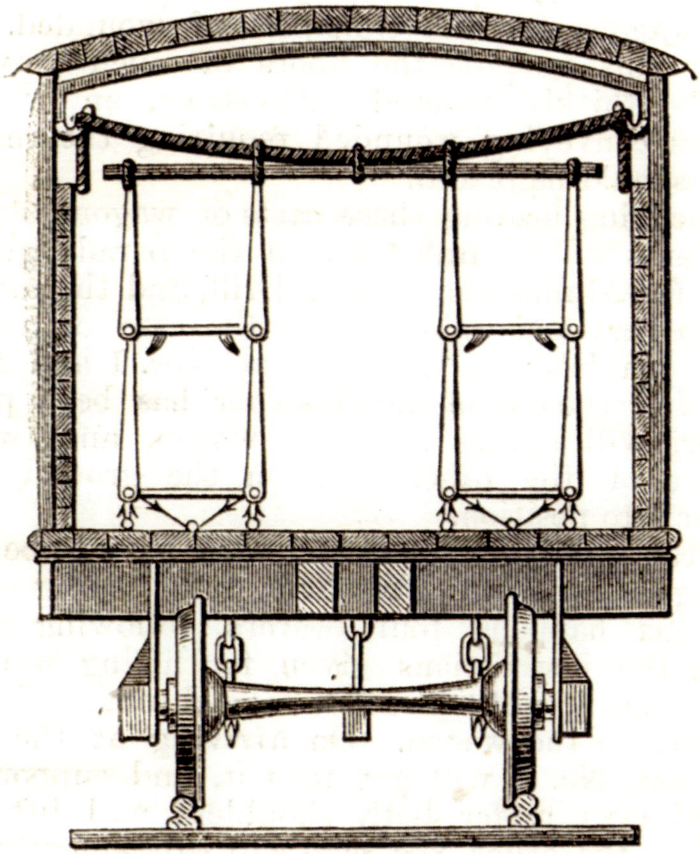

The Zavodovski conversion of a goods wagon.

comprising means of transport, surgical appliances, ambulance and field hospitals, the disposal of the dead and the sanitation of battlefields and encampments'.[7] One of the presentations was from a Russian by the name of Zavodovski, who proposed that in time of war railway goods wagons used to carry troops and stores to the front needed to bring wounded back rather than return empty. He described a system of cables, ropes and ring bolts that could be fitted into a goods wagon in just ten minutes, would carry eight stretchers and cost £3 12*s*. at the time per wagon.[8] By suspending stretchers in this way the hard riding and uncomfortable characteristics of good wagons could be significantly reduced. The Zavodovski conversion was adopted by the British Army and the appropriate drills enshrined in training.

Probably the earliest patient-carrying tramway in Britain was at the Royal Naval Hospital Haslar in Gosport, Hampshire. The hospital opened in 1753 and cared for many thousands of casualties from the Napoleonic Wars along with some 2,000 from the Crimean War.[9] From 1877 patients were transferred in small boats from ships anchored at Spithead and landed at Haslar jetty from where a 400-yard, standard-gauge tramway transferred them to the main hospital building. Two, four-wheeled, hand-propelled ambulance tram cars were built by the Midland Railway Carriage and Wagon Company for this tramway.

Photographs exist of the tramway in use following a fire at Gunwharf on the other side of Portsmouth Harbour in 1910. Casualties were brought across the harbour, landed at Haslar jetty and taken into the hospital on board the ambulance

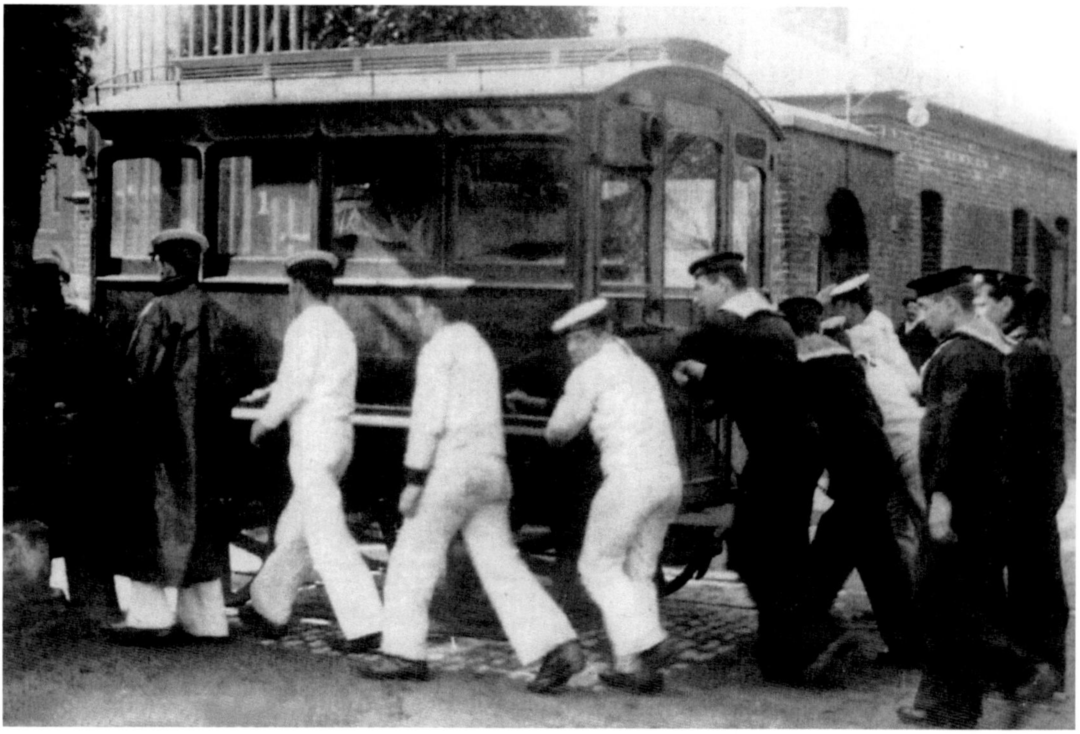

The Royal Naval Hospital Haslar patient-carrying tramway, 1910. (Haslar Heritage Group)

tram cars. The tramway was also used to carry important visitors to the Royal Naval Hospital. King George V and Queen Mary were known to have travelled in one of the ambulance tram cars having arrived at Haslar jetty on an official visit. The tramway was decommissioned in 1920.

The year 1882 saw the Anglo-Egyptian War between Egyptian and Sudanese forces and the British that ultimately led to the British occupation of Egypt. Prior to this there had been a considerable expansion of Egyptian railways largely related to cotton production and its transportation to ports for export. The short campaign between July and September 1882 was of interest in that the arriving British Expeditionary Force made good use of existing Egyptian railway infrastructure but also had the foresight to bring additional railway equipment and some rolling stock by sea.

In a memorandum dated 3 July 1882 Lieutenant General Sir Garnet Wolseley wrote:

> I think I may assume that our operations in the first instance would consist of an advance from Ismailia upon Cairo. A railway passing through Zagazig connects these two places. We may or may not be able to seize some useful amount of rolling stock on that railway, but we should at least make arrangements to be independent, by taking with us 5 locomotives, with large tenders, 5 brake vans, 100 open goods wagons, with tarpaulin covers, and 5 breakdown wagons, with ample supply of tools for repair; also at least 10 miles of steel rails, with bowl sleepers, bolts, nuts, fish-plates, keys, points and crossings in proportions.[10]

This shows the major realisation by British commanders of the value of railways in support of an army in the field. General Wolseley continued in his memorandum that the railway '...will enable us to send our sick daily to the hospital ships at Ismailia'.

In various reports from the campaign there are references to the use of railways to move sick and wounded in the returning empty wagons that had been used for moving stores forward. Clearly how structured this was and whether or not there were dedicated personnel from the Medical Staff Corps to look after the wounded in transit is not known. In a diary entry for 28 August 1882, 21 Company RE were recorded as '...fitting railway trucks as ambulances' at Alexandria. Sadly, no record can be found of the details of the conversion.[11]

The British Army had adopted the Zavodovski conversion to create a casualty carrying capability, but it is not known whether this was used in the Egyptian Campaign or some other local conversion created. The Zavodovski conversion along with all its associated drills were described in the *Manual of the Medical Staff Corps* of 1984.[12] The MSC had been formed in 1855. It was re-organised into the Army Hospital Corps in 1857 but reverted back to its original name in 1884. It subsequently became incorporated into the Royal Army Medical Corps in 1898. The potential to use the Zavodovski conversion continued in the RAMC and could still be found in *Royal Army Medical Corps Training 1908*.[13]

2
South African War

Whilst European countries were embracing the subject of moving casualties by rail it was not the same in Great Britain. In 1898 a paper by Surgeon Major C. H. Melville of the Army Medical Staff was published in the *Royal United Services Institution Journal*.[1] Melville's detailed paper was entitled 'Continental Regulations for the Transport of Sick and Wounded by Rail' and reviewed the use of rail by the German, French, Austrian and Italian armies.

Melville describes the command structures, layout of the trains and their staffing along with the various types of conversions required to carry patients. He presented a wealth of information on what was happening in other countries that is outside the scope of this work but on which future developments in Great Britain could and perhaps should have been based.

At the time Melville was writing British troops had been fighting the Anglo-Zulu War of 1879 in South Africa. There were a number of wars in Southern Africa, but the one usually referred to as the South African War, Second Boer War or the Anglo-Boer War was fought between October 1899 and 31 May 1902. It was fought between the British Empire and the Boer republics of the Transvaal and the Orange Free State. Rail was to play an important part in this war not only for the movement of men, stores and ammunition but both sides ran what were referred to at the time as hospital trains.

During the South African War four different types of hospital trains were utilised by the British. Firstly, seven trains were converted from locally available rolling stock. One purpose-built train, the Princess Christian Hospital Train, was shipped out from England. There were also a number of improvised trains that were unconverted local rolling stock used for less serious cases. Finally, there were single ambulance coaches that were converted to take lying and sitting patients. They were strategically placed, used to pick up small groups of casualties and then attached to other trains for conveyance to the nearest hospital. Very little detail survives about these coaches, but one NCO and one orderly staffed each coach with medical officers from units along the route assisting where necessary.

No. 1 Hospital Train was prepared by Natal Government Railways in Durban in September 1899. It consisted of ordinary passenger stock with very little modification and was ready for use by the outbreak of hostilities. There was no through corridor. Of note is that the doorways were unaltered and special narrow stretchers were apparently used to load casualties.[2]

No. 1A Hospital Train was similar to No. 1 and also prepared by Natal Government Railways in Durban and completed by December 1899.

No. 2 Hospital Train was prepared at Cape Town in September 1899. It was converted from a mixture of passenger and post office rolling stock and carried ninety-six lying patients. This train was staffed by personnel from England.

No. 3 Hospital Train was also converted in Cape Town. It only carried ninety-two lying patients also staffed by personnel from England.

No. 4 Hospital Train was converted at East London at the expense of the British Red Cross. Work commenced on the train in April 1900 and it undertook its first journey on 10 June 1900. The dining and kitchen cars were supplied by the Orange Free State Railways. The train consisted of five ward coaches giving a capacity of seventy-two lying patients. It was a continuous corridor train and had a toilet in each coach. The train was painted white with Red Cross emblems on the sides prior

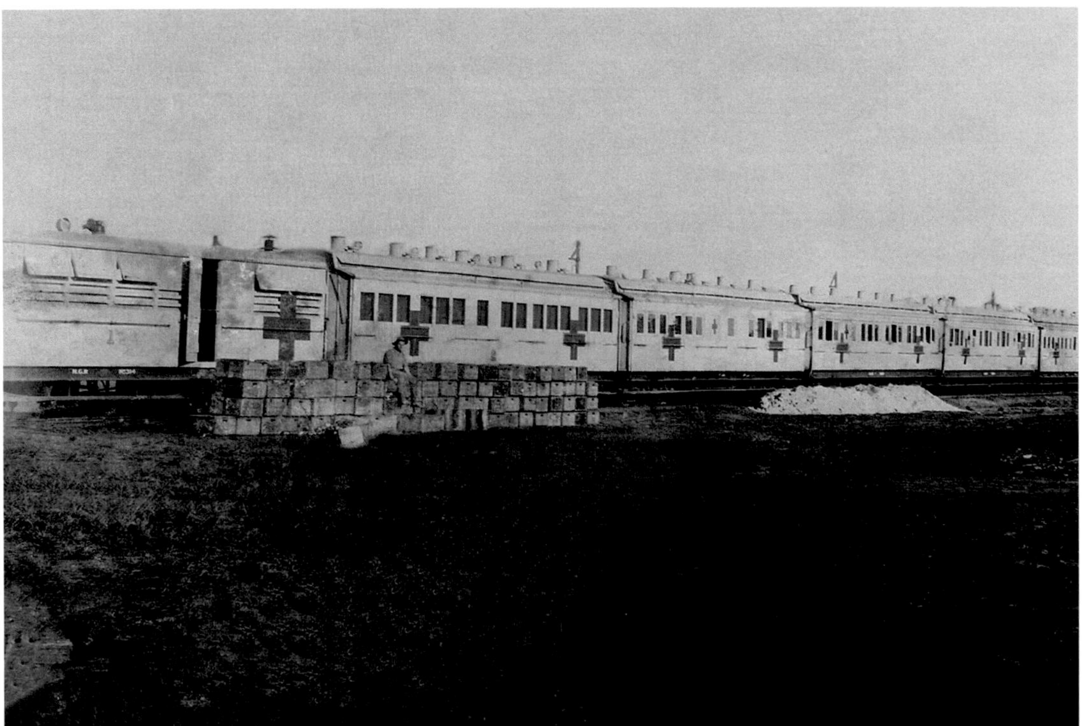

A digitally enhanced photograph of a Natal Government Railways hospital train at Howich Hospital during the South African War.

to entering service. After deployment further vans were added for stores and two further coaches were added increasing the patient capacity to 114.[3]

No. 5 Hospital Train was prepared at Cape Town and consisted of seven converted Cape Government Railways passenger coaches and carried ninety-two lying patients.

No. 6 Hospital Train was an abandoned Boer train about which little detail has survived.

On 18 October 1899 a contract was signed by Sir John Furley on behalf of the Central Committee of the British Red Cross and by Mr W. J. Fieldhouse for the Military Equipment Committee for the provision of a purpose-built hospital train for service in South Africa.[4] This was funded by the British Red Cross along with the Borough of Windsor, Berkshire and other benefactors. This was a seven-coach train and was constructed by the Birmingham Railway Carriage and Wagon Company. It was named after the Princess Christian of Schleswig-Holstein, who was the fifth child of Queen Victoria.[5] She was also a founder member of the British Red Cross which had been created from the British Society for Aid to the Sick and Wounded in War that had been formed in 1870.

The train was completed ahead of schedule in just ten weeks. It was of wooden construction and had seven bogie corridor coaches, each 36 ft long.[6] Once complete, it was deconstructed and in effect 'flat packed' and shipped out to Durban, arriving on 7 March 1900 where after reconstruction it entered service on 17 May 1900.

The train was designed to accommodate seventy-four lying patients (two officers and seventy-two men) with a staff that consisted of two medical officers, two nursing sisters, one cook, one compounder (a pharmacist of the day) and twelve orderlies.

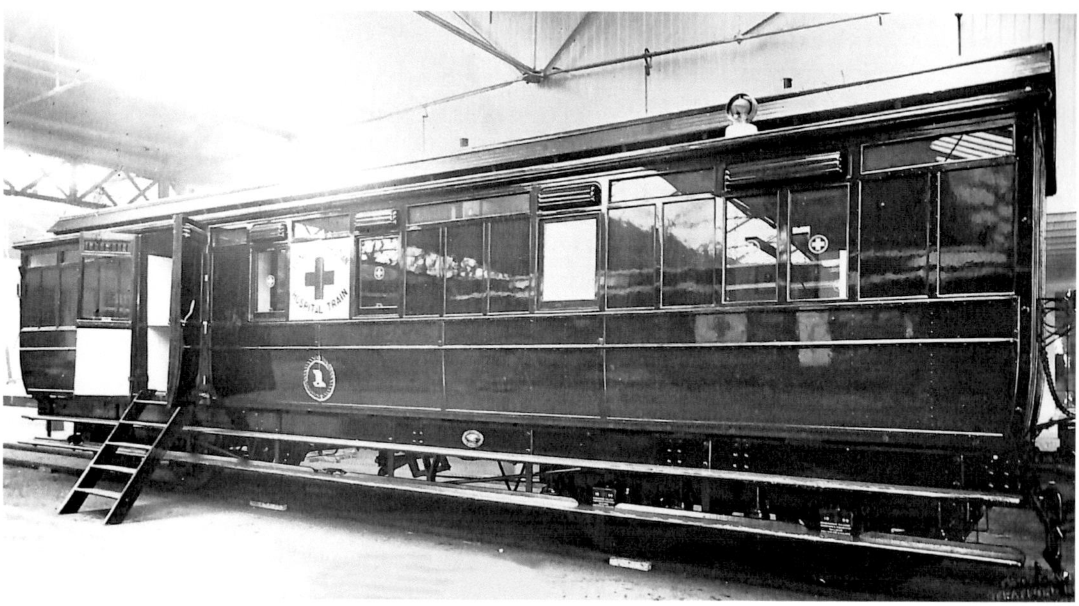

Exterior view of a carriage from the Princess Christian Hospital Train. (British Red Cross Museum and Archives)

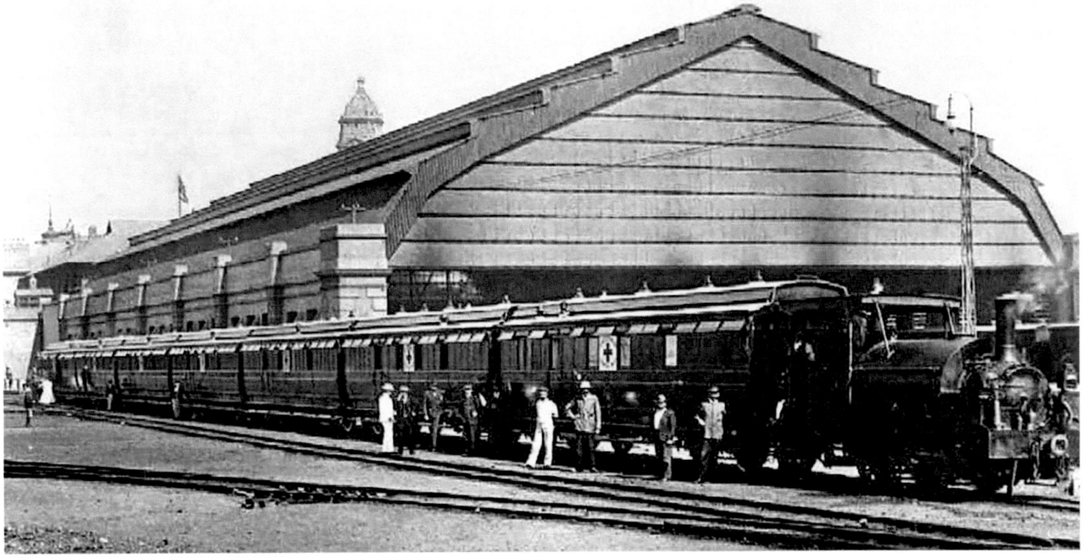

The Princess Christian Hospital Train at Durban in 1900 prior to deployment. (Alamy)

The layout of the seven coaches was as follows. Coach 1 contained three sections namely stores, accommodation for two nurses and for two sick or wounded officers. Coach 2 also had three sections namely accommodation for two medical officers, the dining room and dispensary. Coaches 3, 4, 5 and 6 had accommodation for eighteen patients along with four hospital orderlies each. Coach 7 contained the kitchen, accommodation for two cooks and a compartment for the train guard.

On the outside of each coach a central panel carried the Red Cross emblem surrounded by 'Princess Christian Hospital Train' in royal blue and gold. The train also carried the Union Jack and Red Cross flags on the front of the train.

History tells us that the first trip of the train was as part of the force sent to relieve the siege of Ladysmith. When it reached the Tugela River on 19 March the construction of the trestle bridge for the railway had not been completed. As soon as the work was finished the train proceeded into Ladysmith. Between 20 and 26 March 1900 the Princess Christian Hospital Train's first four journeys were the removal of sick and wounded from Ladysmith and transporting them on three trips direct to Durban and a fourth trip to Mooi River that continued to Durban.[7]

Much correspondence came back from South Africa to Lord Wantage (1832–1901) who was a co-founder and first chairman of the British Red Cross. One letter from the assistant commissioner of the Red Cross, Gerald Bonham-Carter, refers to the Princess Christian Hospital Train.[8] On 30 December 1900 he wrote:

> At the beginning of August the train was sent down to Durban for repairs. It was thoroughly overhauled and painted white from end to end with large Red Crosses at intervals making it very conspicuous... The short carriages and bogie wheels of the Princess Christian Hospital Train make it particularly well suited to the sharp curves of the Komati Poort line.

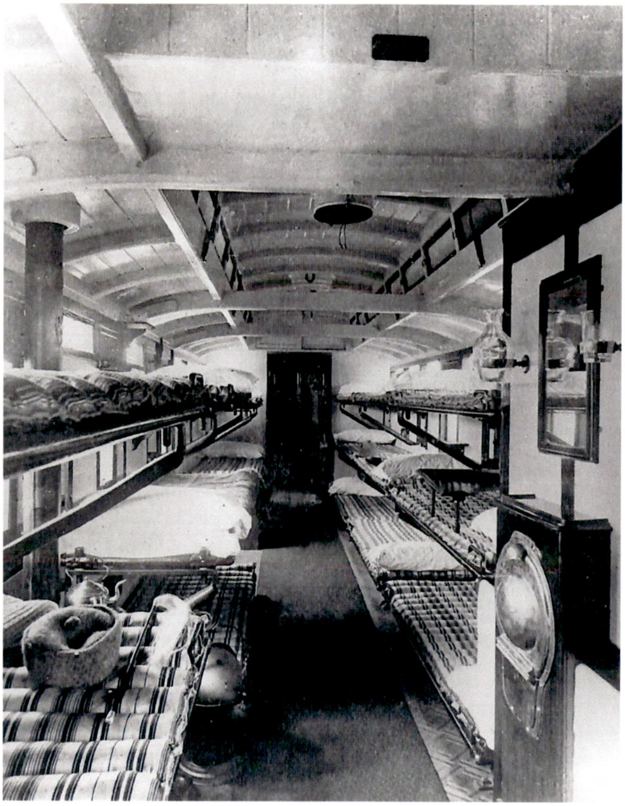

Ward accommodation on the Princess Christian Hospital Train. (British Red Cross Museum and Archives)

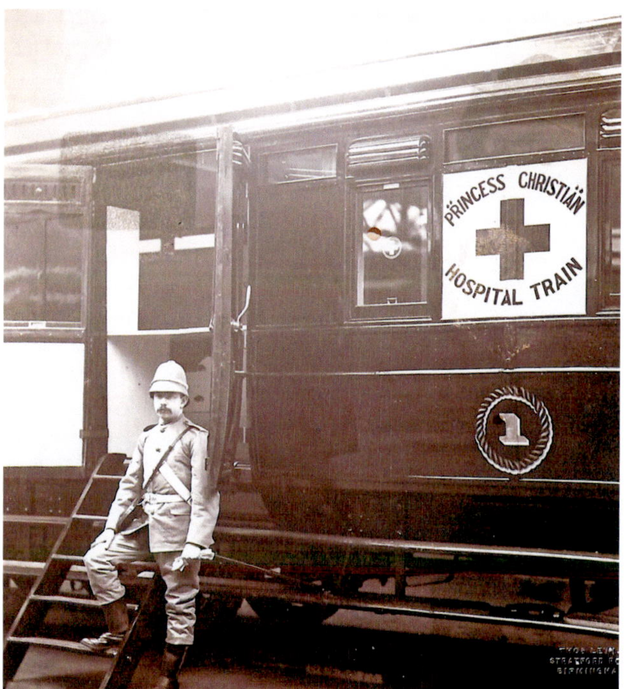

The Princess Christian Hospital Train before deployment. (British Red Cross Museum and Archives)

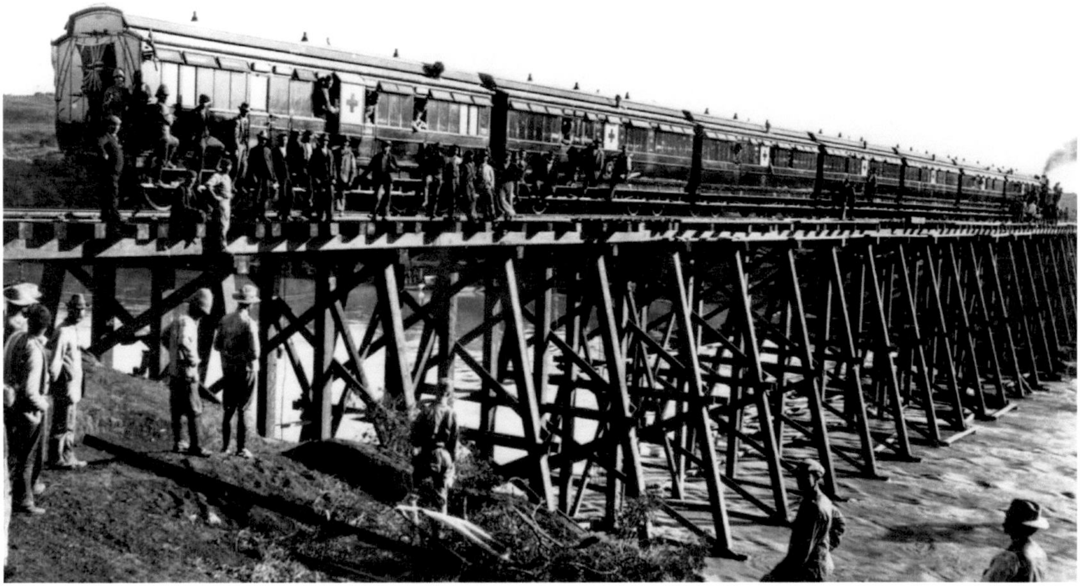

The Princess Christian Hospital Train crossing the Teluga River on 19 March 1900.

Details of the 108 journeys undertaken by the train and lists of routes, dates and casualty loads of each are contained in a British Red Cross Report. The train travelled some 42,115 miles and carried a total of 7,548 patients. Records show that there were just three deaths amongst the patients carried along with three deaths amongst train staff.[9]

Reference was made earlier to the fact that staff for Nos 2 and 3 Hospital Trains, along with the staff for the Princess Christian Hospital Train sailed out from England. These would have included RAMC personnel and nursing sisters. The Army Nursing Service was raised in 1861 and the Army Nursing Service Reserve in 1897. At the commencement of the South African War the ANSR had 101 nursing sisters, and a number were to serve in the hospitals and on the hospital trains. What is not so widely known is that 2,046 men from St John Ambulance served in South Africa and provided almost a quarter of the entire medical manpower during the campaign.[10] It is also of interest that they deployed wearing khaki uniforms whereas British soldiers in South Africa were in the main still wearing red tunics. In addition, there were also locally engaged medical and nursing personnel along with civilian surgeons from England. The term civilian surgeon was used at the time to refer to any doctor rather than a specialist in surgery.

Some 500 civilian surgeons were appointed and served during the campaign. The Royal Commission that looked into the care of sick and wounded during the South African War recorded that 'Civilian surgeons employed in the campaign have, as a body, done their duty extremely well.'[11] Of interest, several of the doctors who served as civilian surgeons went on to become famous in various branches of medicine, surgery and literature. Two such individuals were Sir Frederick Treves and Sir Arthur Conan Doyle.

The operating of trains, for whatever purpose, required two important commodities: coal and water. One of the early battles of the war was the Battle of Talana Hill in Natal, also variously referred to as the Battle of Glencoe or the Battle of Dundee. It took place on 20 October 1899 and was a British victory, although with heavy losses. Lying between Talana Hill and Glencoe was the mining town of Dundee, which was of strategic importance to the British as a source of coal for the steam locomotives that pulled hospital and other military trains. The line ran from Dundee to Glencoe Junction, which was on the main line from Johannesburg to Durban via Ladysmith. Dundee was also the location of No. 40 Stationary Hospital, which was a 100-bed hospital that was operational between 12 October 1900 and 31 May 1902.[12]

Mention should also be made that the Boers also operated ambulance trains. Of major importance to the Boers was the Netherlands South African Railway which had created the railway network in the Transvaal. In particular, the railway provided access to Lourenço Marques, a port not under British control.[13] Foreign medical and nursing volunteers supporting the Boer cause came from several countries including Belgium, Germany, France and America. It is known that Dutch and Russian nurses served on Boer ambulance trains.

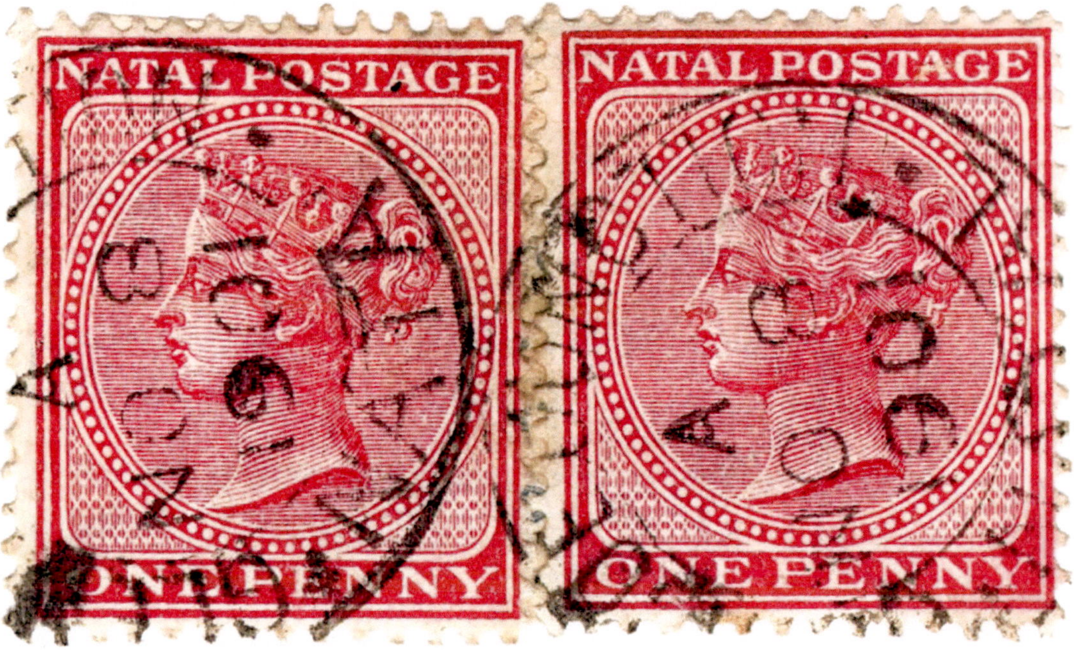

A pair of Natal 1*d.* stamps carrying the cancellation of 'GLENCOE JUNCTION NATAL' dated 8 November 1901.

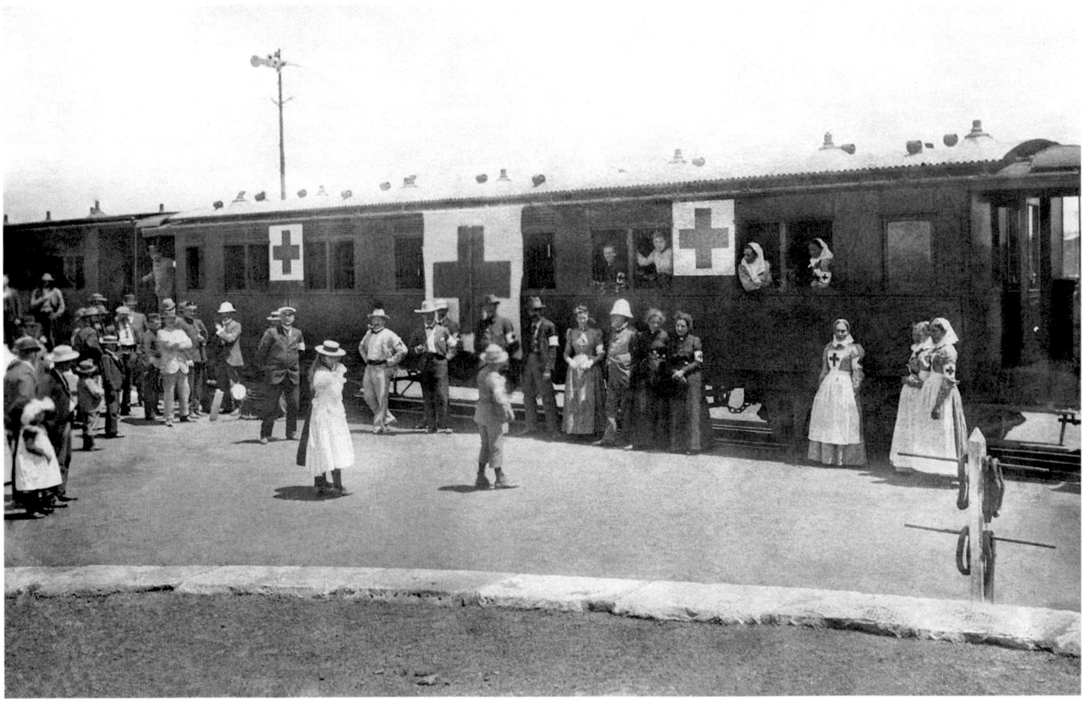

A digitally enhanced photograph of a Boer hospital train at Lourenço Marques in former Portuguese East Africa.

The return of the sick and wounded from the South African War to Great Britain was by hospital trains from the various hospitals to a port and then by hospital ships, the history of which is a major subject in its own right. Ten ships were converted to transport casualties back to Great Britain with the usual embarkation ports being Durban or Cape Town. Some of the ships also provided temporary hospital facilities at anchor in Durban Harbour.

A photograph survives showing the SS *Lismore Castle* with an unidentified hospital train standing alongside. This ship was built in 1891 in Scotland and was operated by the Union-Castle Mail Steamship Company. It sailed from Southampton on 20 October 1899 and arrived at Cape Town in South Africa on 11 November 1899. It subsequently moved to Durban for conversion to a hospital ship with a patient capacity of 214, which was completed on 9 December 1899. The SS *Lismore Castle* and several other converted ships were not declared under the Geneva Convention and therefore did not display the Red Cross emblem. This was because they were used to carry troops on their return trips. In this latter role the SS *Lismore Castle* became known as *Troop Ship No. 28*.[14]

Most of the wounded from the South African War returned to the Royal Victoria Hospital, Netley, Hampshire, whose foundation stone had been laid by Queen Victoria in May 1856. It was a very large imposing building some quarter of a mile in length on the banks of Southampton Water. It was to become the largest military hospital in Great Britain, with 138 wards containing approximately 1,000 beds and

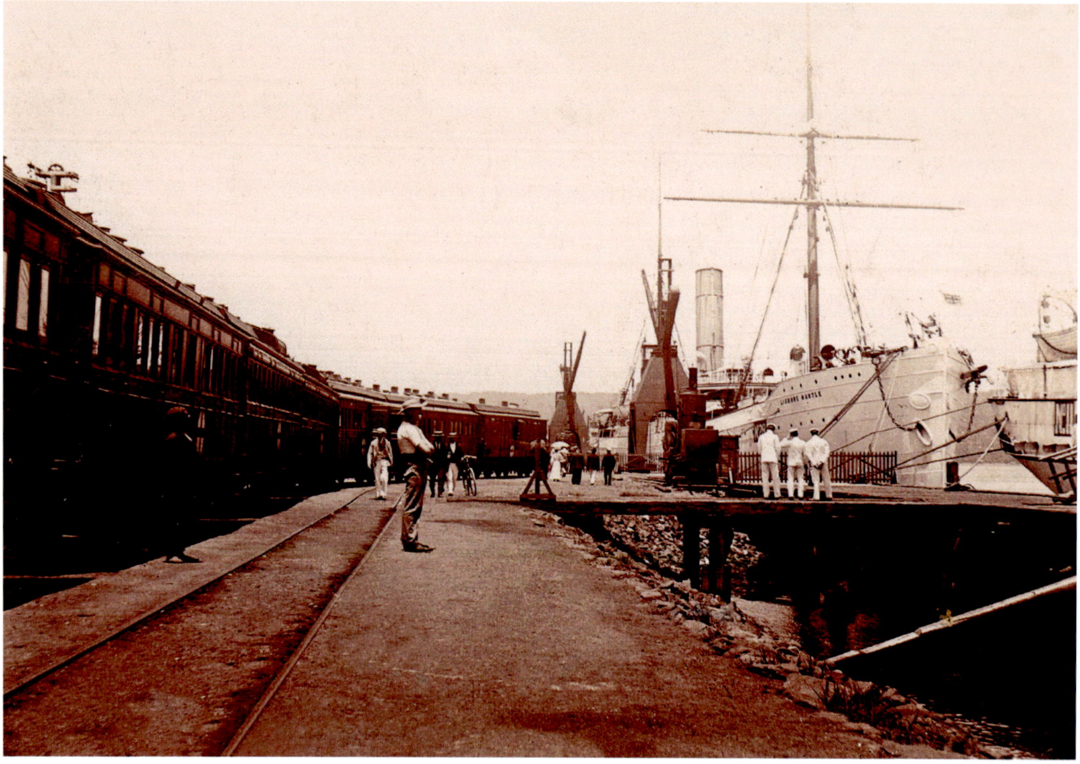

An unidentified hospital train alongside SS *Lismore Castle*, likely to be at Durban.

it received its first patients on 11 March 1863. Sick and wounded were returned to Southampton in hospital ships from campaigns including India in 1865, Sudan in 1882 and Egypt in 1885.[15] Casualties arriving at Southampton Docks needed to travel by rail because the hospital jetty did not reach far enough out into deep water in order to accommodate large hospital ships.

Netley Railway Station was originally opened in 1866 and the presence of such a large hospital turned this quiet village station into the third busiest railway station in the country at the time.[16] In 1899 a decision was made to build a branch directly into the hospital grounds and establish a Hospital Station.

The *London & South Western Railway Instruction No. 17 of 1900* carries a description of the opening of the new line between Netley Station and the Royal Victoria Hospital that took place on 18 April 1900.[17] It was a single-line branch that would only be operated as required for the running of ambulance trains. The loop line at the Hospital Station gave 650 ft of clear standing space and there was one platform 196 ft in length.

During the latter stages of the South African War the LSWR converted five 48-ft fruit vans into ambulance coaches. These formed the War Department ambulance train, but the coaches became more commonly known simply as 'Netley' coaches. They were stored on the Netley Hospital branch line and were used to transfer patients arriving at Southampton direct to the hospital.

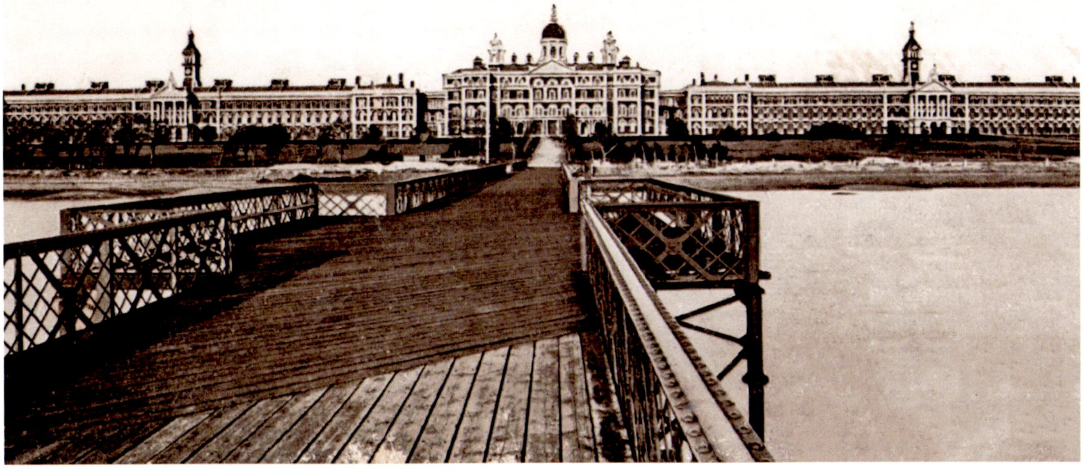

A postcard of the Royal Victoria Hospital, Netley, showing its jetty.

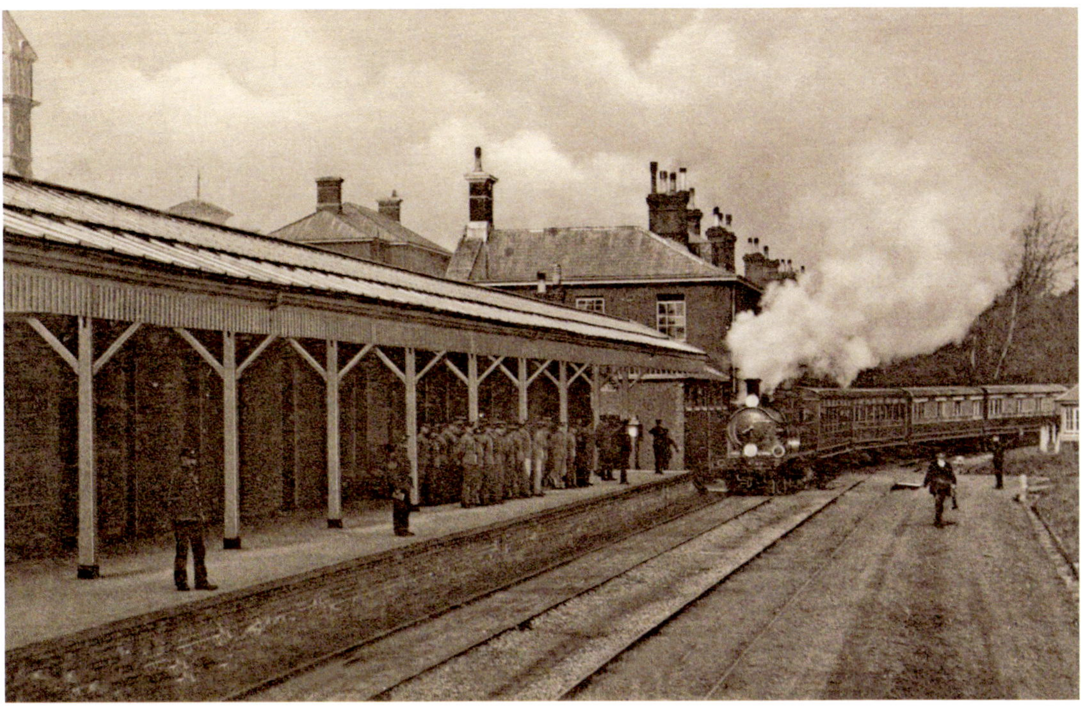

A postcard showing a train arriving at the Royal Victoria Hospital Station.

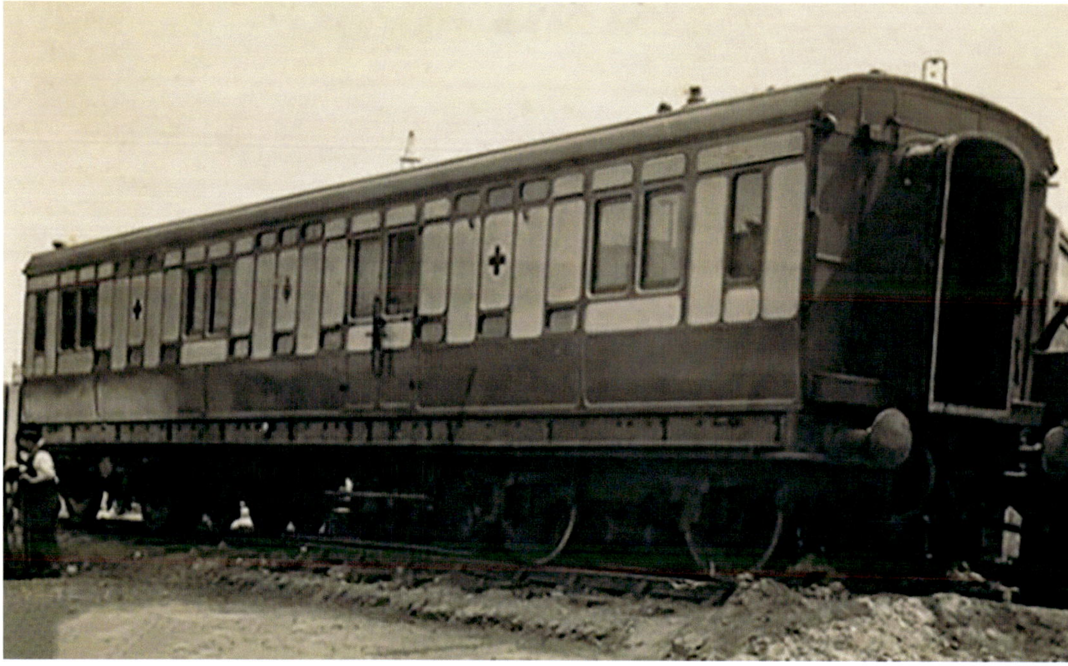

One of the five 'Netley' coaches that formed the War Department Ambulance Train. (Museum of Military Medicine. Ref: L0070596)

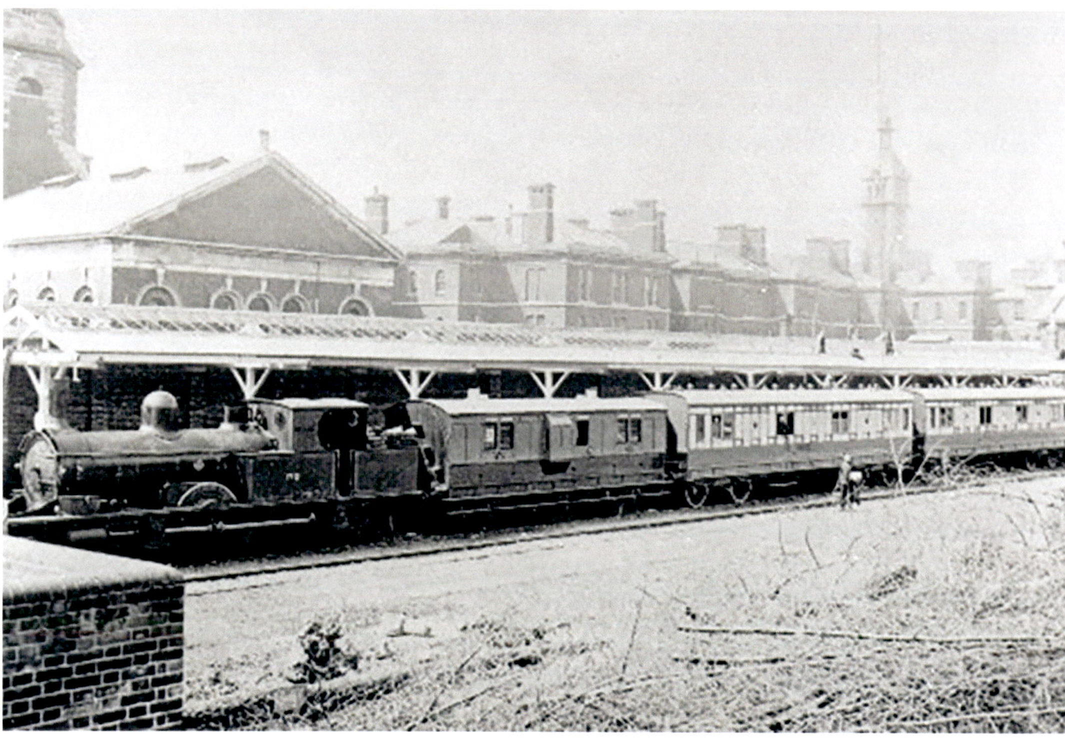

The War Department Ambulance Train at the Royal Victoria Hospital Station in 1900.

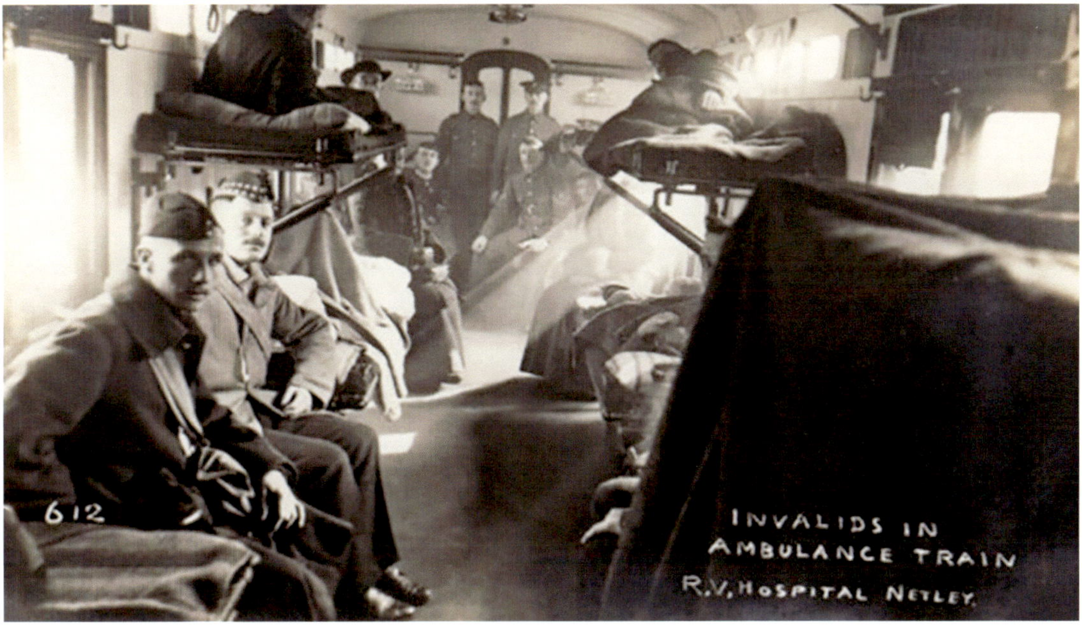

A postcard showing patients inside one of the 'Netley' coaches.

Over 75,000 sick and wounded were returned home from the South African War. Over 26,000 British troops along with over 40,000 civilians died during the war.[18] The war was ended by the Treaty of Vereeniging that was signed on 31 May 1902. The treaty placed the two Boer republics back within the British Empire and the Union of South Africa was eventually established within the British Empire in 1910.

Several reports, including a Royal Commission, enquired into the care provided to the sick and wounded of the South African War. That there were deficiencies in manpower, resources and care are recorded in many sources but some comments specifically about trains are pertinent. The Royal Commission stated: 'Special praise should also be given to the authorities in respect of ambulance trains, which were largely used in the campaign and with excellent results.'[19]

The *British Medical Journal* of 1903 also carried evidence about the medical services during the war. The evidence of one eminent physician of the time, Professor Ogston, is quoted and included:

> They had trains for the wounded, and they had trains for the sick and what he saw in South Africa convinced him that it was of the utmost importance that there should be trains for fever. He thought that if the question of sick transport has been well thought out beforehand it could have been better done in South Africa. The trains in South Africa were as well done as care and zeal could manage, but they were not what they should have been.[20]

A decade later in the First World War the Austro-Hungarian Empire did exactly what was suggested and produced *Infektionskrankenzüge* (ambulance trains for infectious patients) which served specific infectious disease hospitals.

3
First World War

Wednesday, October 14th – still in the siding waiting for orders to move. There's a lot of waiting to be done in this War one way and another, as well as a lot of doing.

K. E. Luard[1]

Between the South African War and the First World War the British changed the name of its trains from hospital to ambulance trains. During the First World War there were both home and overseas ambulance trains. Ambulance trains were operated by the Royal Navy, the Friends' Ambulance Unit, as well as American forces after they had entered the war. Ambulance trains were also used in other theatres of the war such as Salonika, Mesopotamia and East Africa.

HOME AMBULANCE TRAINS

At the outbreak of the First World War only the War Department Ambulance Train consisting of 'Netley' coaches was available for use. The first casualties from the British Expeditionary Force (BEF) arrived at Southampton Docks on 24 August 1914 and were transferred to the Royal Victoria Hospital, Netley, in this train.

At the outbreak of war an initial order for twelve HATs was placed. These first twelve trains were produced from various railway companies as follows: three from the LNWR, two each from the GCR, GWR and MR along with one each from the GER, the LYR and the LSWR.[2] They were of nine vehicles in length, of which five were ward coaches converted to carry twenty patients each. Each train also had coaches for pharmacy, office and stores, kitchen and staff accommodation. This first tranche of HATs retained their individual company liveries with the addition of the Red Cross to the roof and sides. The HATs were staffed by a medical officer, two

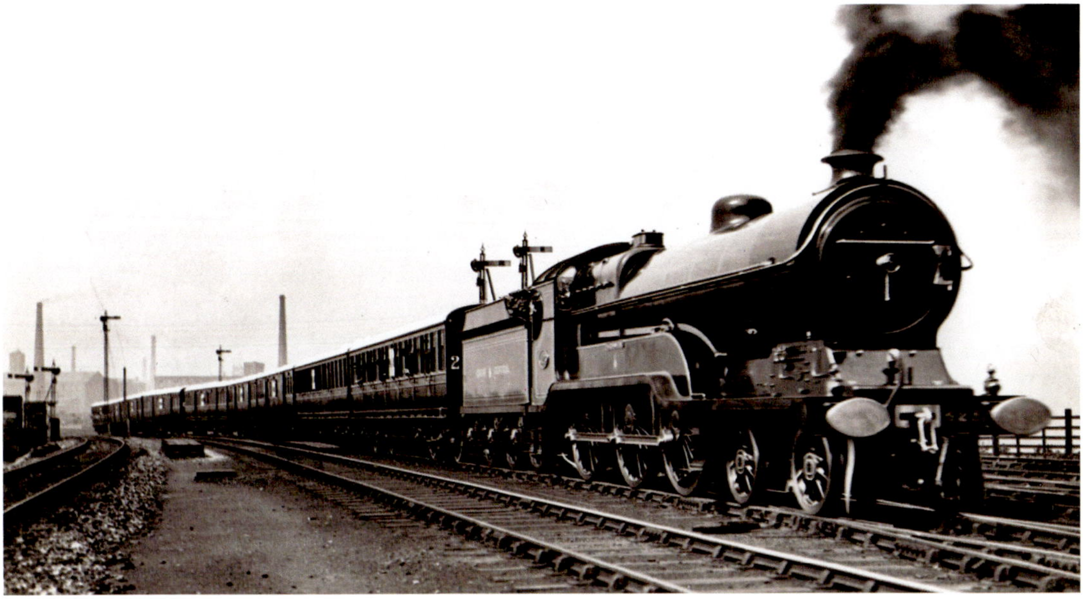

Great Central Railway No. 2 (Home) Ambulance Train. (© The Board of Trustees of the Science Museum, Ref: LNER RO/129)

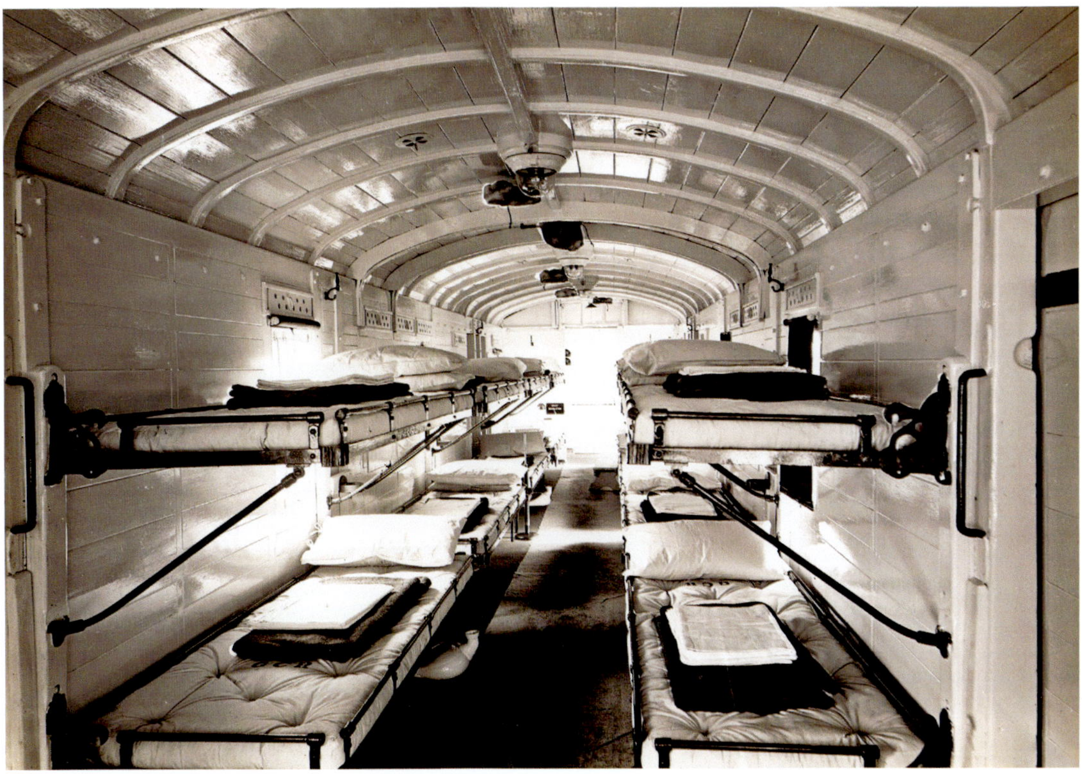

Interior of a ward coach of either No. 1 or No. 2 (Home) Ambulance Train. (© The Board of Trustees of the Science Museum, Ref: LNER RO/206)

nursing sisters and twelve RAMC other ranks with catering staff provided by the company supplying the rolling stock.

Mention should be made that the NER contributed a number of 25-ton vans converted to take twelve stretcher patients each. These somewhat spartan conversions were initially used to collect casualties at north-eastern ports and, by being coupled to scheduled trains, distribute them around hospitals in York and its environs.

The early returning casualties from the BEF were distributed to existing military hospitals but the need for beds rapidly increased to utilise civilian, auxiliary and private hospitals along with ever increasing numbers of convalescent homes. Plumridge tells us that at the outbreak of the war there were 7,000 beds available in military hospitals, but this rose to a total of 364,133 in hospitals of all types all across the country.[3] Some 196 railway stations around Great Britain are recorded as receiving ambulance trains during the course of the First World War.[4]

In January 1915 the War Office requested a further four ambulance trains and these were provided by the GCR, GWR, LYR and LNWR. At about the same time a decision was made that each of the sixteen HATs should have the addition of two corridor coaches for sitting casualties. Five emergency ambulance trains were also commissioned that consisted of standard corridor coaches along with a dining car. These trains were only intended for sitting casualties and initially allocated to Dover and Southampton.[5] Four more HATs were also produced by the LNWR, GWR, GER and LSWR, bringing the total to twenty.

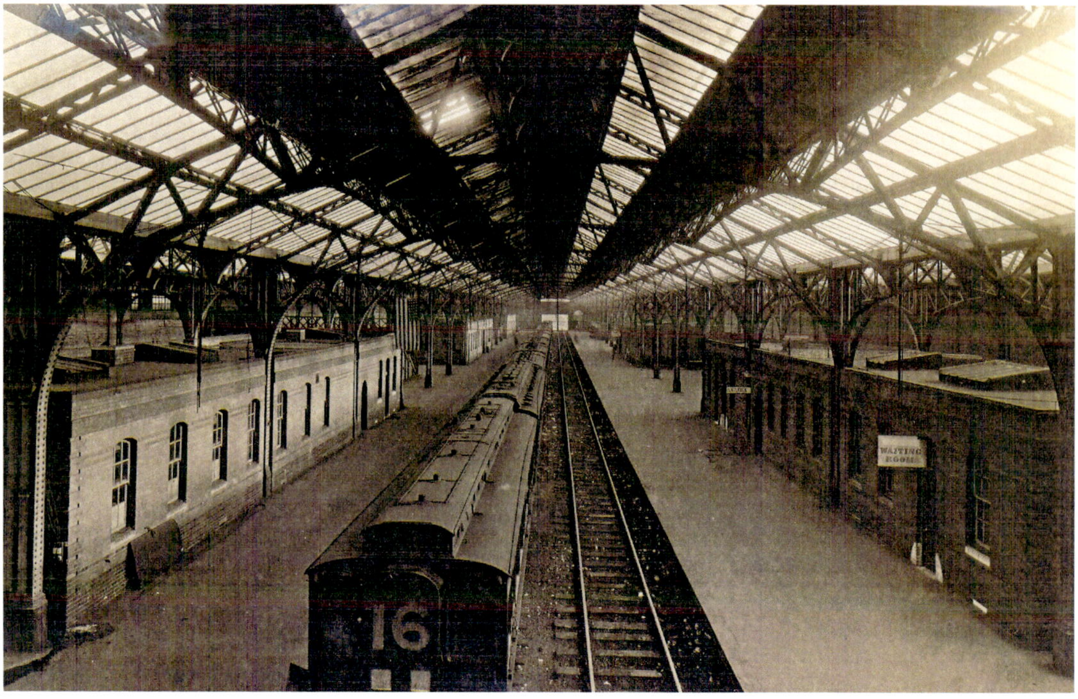

No. 16 (Home) Ambulance Train at Dover Marine Station. (R. J. E. Bayliff Collection)

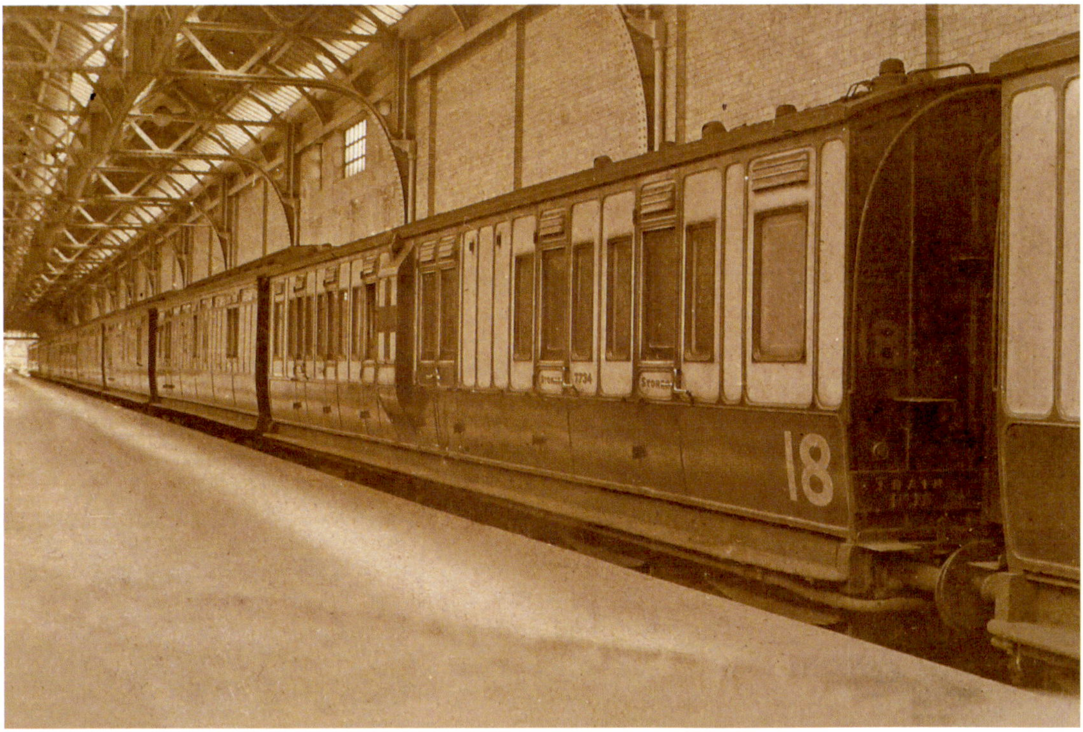

No. 18 (Home) Ambulance Train at Southampton Docks.

Home ambulance trains were under the overall command of Central Force, which was the Home Command of the British Army during the First World War. Formed on 5 August 1914 Central Force had its HQ in London with the First Army HQ in Bedford, the Second Army in Aldershot and the Third Army in Luton.

Specific control of ambulance trains and the distribution of casualties was initially from Southampton. In 1917 the scale of operations was such that a decision was made to move the HQ to Adastral House in London.[6] From here, bed availability throughout the country was monitored. Efforts were made to send casualties to hospitals near their homes and there were also specific hospitals for Canadian, Australian, Indian and troops from other countries.

Ambulance trains were also used to transfer patients between hospitals as their care dictated and it was not unusual for a train to stop simply to take on or set down a single patient. The level of planning for each ambulance train journey was considerable and was well described by the following example from a train departing Dover, reproduced as published.[7]

> Ambulance boat, Jan Breydel. Due 2.30 pm. Berth No 2. Number of ambulance train 16. To convey Canadians to Taplow (Great Western Railway), and thence to Temple Meads, Bristol, with 100 cot and 60 sitting cases, together with three cot patients picked up at Addison Road for transfer to Temple Meads. On the return journey, stop at Taplow to set down five cot Canadians and at Addison Road to set down one cot case, all from Temple Meads.

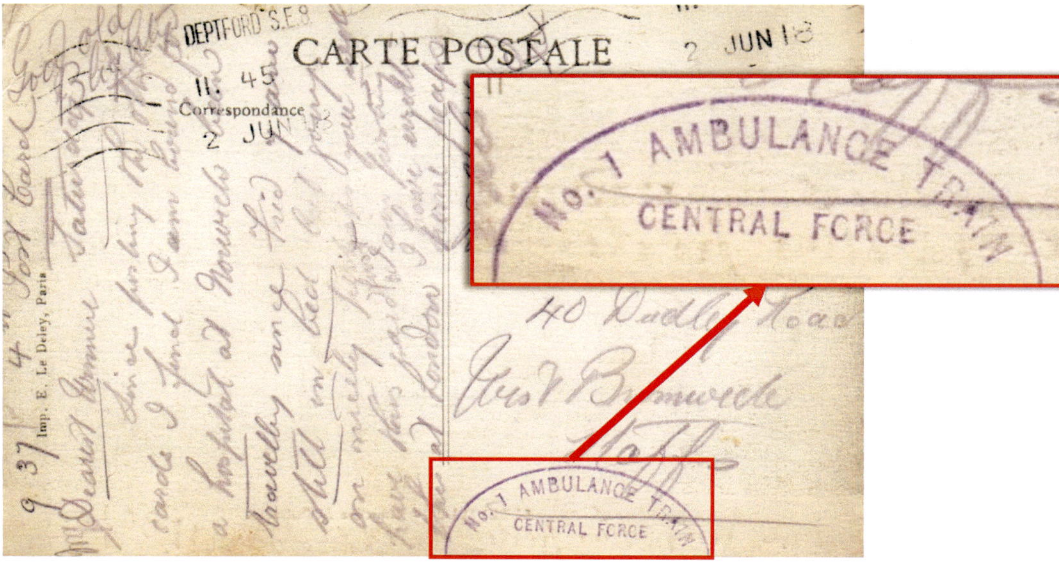

A postcard posted from Deptford in south-east London in June 1918 carrying the handstamp of 'No. 1 AMBULANCE TRAIN CENTRAL FORCE'.

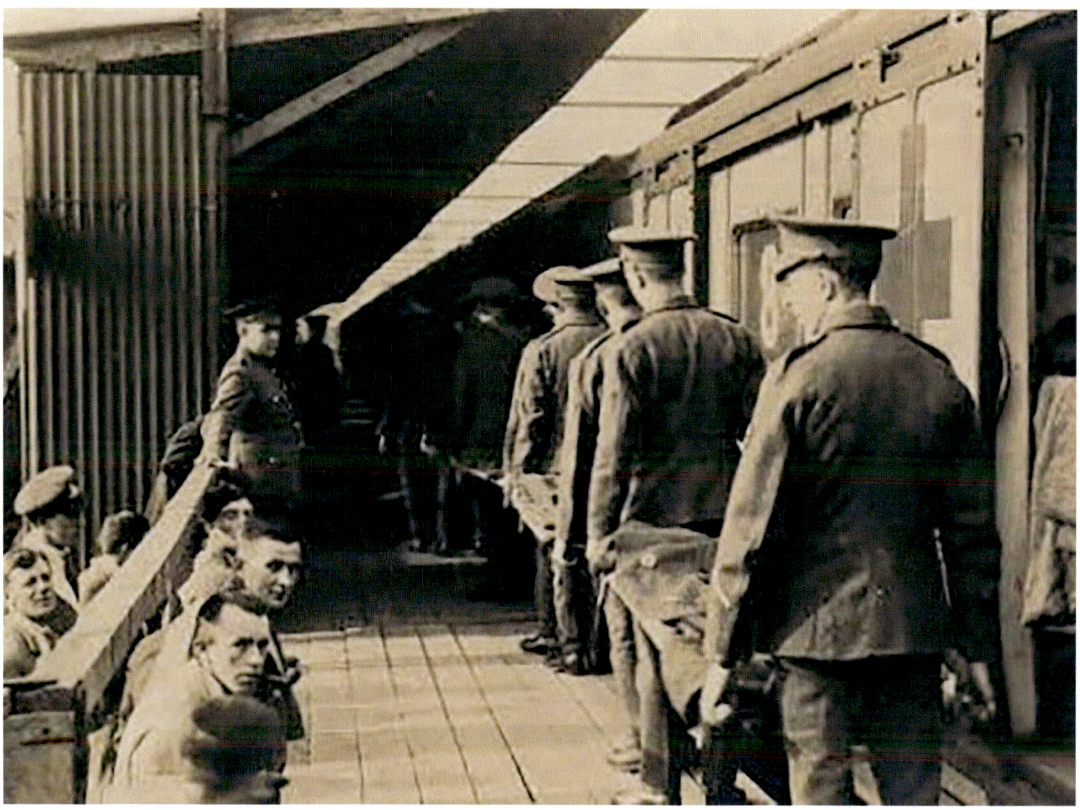

A postcard showing patients being unloaded at the Queen Mary's Military Hospital Station at Whalley, Lancashire, in 1917.

Southampton and Dover were the main ports from which ambulance trains operated in order to distribute casualties around the country. However, other ports were used including Avonmouth, Devonport, Liverpool, Leith, Hull and Boston. The Port of London was also used occasionally.[8]

Several statistics illustrate the major contribution the HATs made to the war effort. A total of 7,822 ambulance train journeys distributed some 1,250,000 casualties who had arrived at Southampton Docks alone between 24 August 1914 and 31 December 1918.[9] The new Dover Marine Station did not become fully operational until into 1915, by which time it was possible for two hospital ships and six ambulance trains to be handled at the same time.[10] For Dover, history records that 4,076 hospital ship journeys delivered some 1,260,506 casualties between 2 January 1915 and 28 February 1919. These required some 7,781 ambulance train journeys to distribute them around the country.[11]

ROYAL NAVY (HOME) AMBULANCE TRAINS

Early in the war the Admiralty formed the Naval Medical Transport Service to manage the reception of Royal Navy casualties at the major naval ports. This service was planned by Surgeon General Sir James Porter KCB, RN, who divided the coastal areas of the country into five areas, with Scotland being the most important. The others had their HQs at Chatham, Portsmouth, Plymouth and Hull.[12] Five Royal Naval ambulance trains were integral to the service and ensured collection of disembarked casualties and their distribution to naval hospitals around the country. Details of the five RN ambulance trains can be found in the table below.

Train Number	Stock	Date Completed	Coaches	First Run Date
RN Ambulance Train No. 1	LNWR	August 1914	13	17 September 1914
RN Ambulance Train No. 2	LNWR	June 1915	12	22 June 1915
RN Ambulance Train No. 3	LNWR	June 1916	12	2 June 1916 **
RN Ambulance Train No. 4	LNWR	June 1916	7	9 June 1916
RN Ambulance Train No. 5	LNWR	March 1918	12	21 March 1918
** On display to the public at Addison Road Station, London, 11 and 12 June 1916				

A sixth train was commissioned in September 1918. However, with the war ending the order was cancelled in December 1918, with only two coaches having been converted.[13]

The first of these ambulance trains was completed at Wolverton Carriage Works in Buckinghamshire on 8 August 1914 and dispatched to Chatham Dockyard. Four of these Royal Naval trains, Numbers 1, 2, 3 and 5, operated between Scotland and England. Two of the trains were based in Craigentinny carriage sidings, Edinburgh,

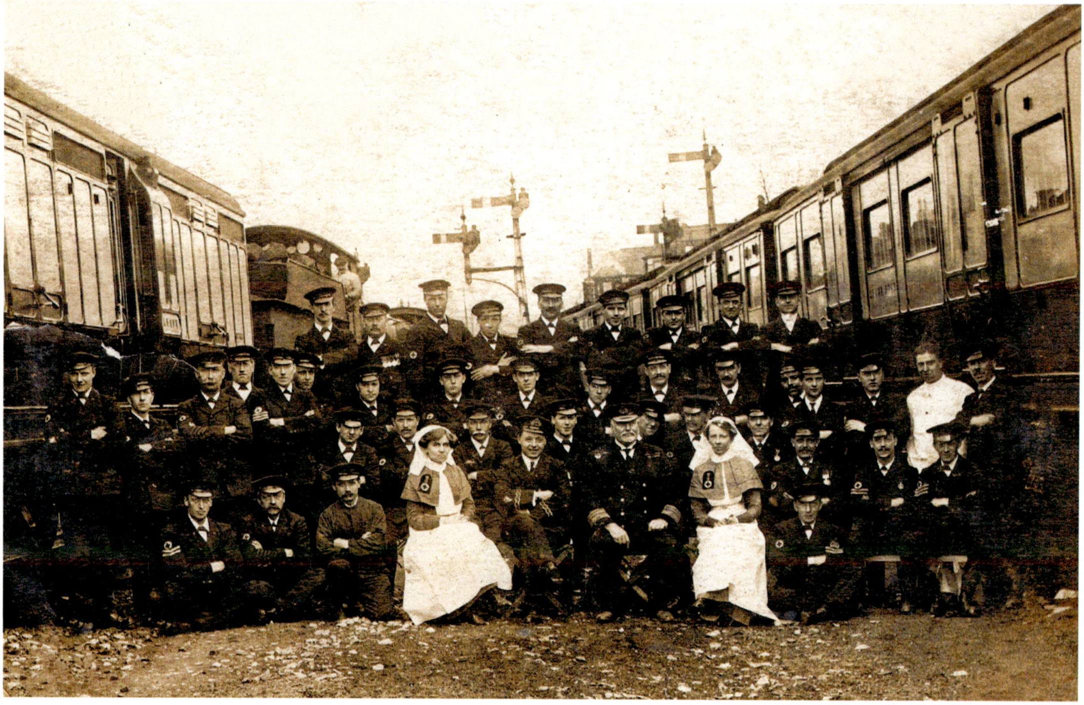

RN ambulance train staff assumed to be at Chatham. The senior staff are detailed on the reverse, which included the Surgeon General Sir James Porter, who was known to have been at Chatham when the first RN train was delivered.

with one each at Dawsholm, Glasgow and Chatham Dockyard in Kent. These were, however, interchangeable and operated around hospitals in the central belt of Scotland. There were then workings down the east coast ports, including Hull and Boston and then on to Plymouth, Gosport and terminating in Chatham Dockyard. RN Ambulance Train No. 4 had a shorter length of only seven coaches and was based in Inverness. It remained within Scotland operating around the Highland Line working from the ports of Invergordon and Thurso.

The Royal Navy ambulance trains were painted grey and carried port and starboard labels as if they were ships. The staff of a RN ambulance train consisted of two medical officers, two QARNNS nursing officers and thirty-six Royal Naval Auxiliary Sick Berth Reserve personnel and they operated standard sea watches as if based on a warship.[14]

The major difference between the RN ambulance trains and those operated by the Army was that the patient was carried in a cot. This was both a bed and a stretcher and once placed in it on the ship the wounded sailor stayed in it throughout their journey. Within the ambulance trains the cots were suspended from the roof and free to swing as a hammock. Each ward coach carried twenty-four cots.

Shown in the table above RN Ambulance Train No. 3 was opened to the public at Addison Road (now Kensington Olympia) Station in London on 11 and 12 June 1916. The admission charge to view the train was 1*s*. (current equivalent: 5p) with

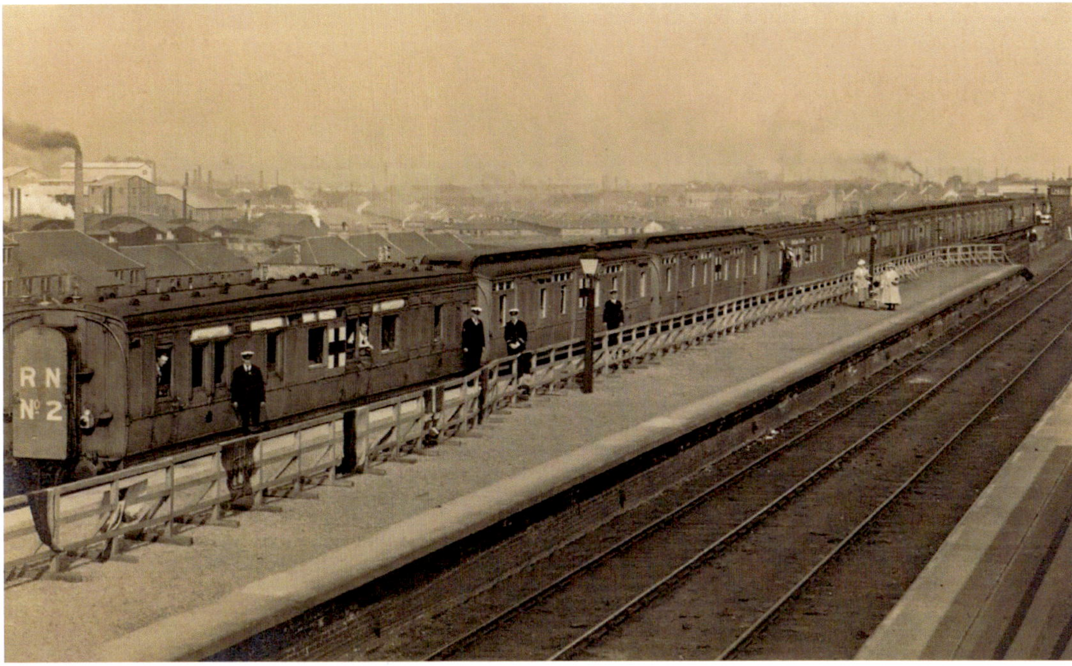

A postcard showing RN (Home) Ambulance Train No. 2 at Wishaw Station, North Lanarkshire, Scotland, in 1918.

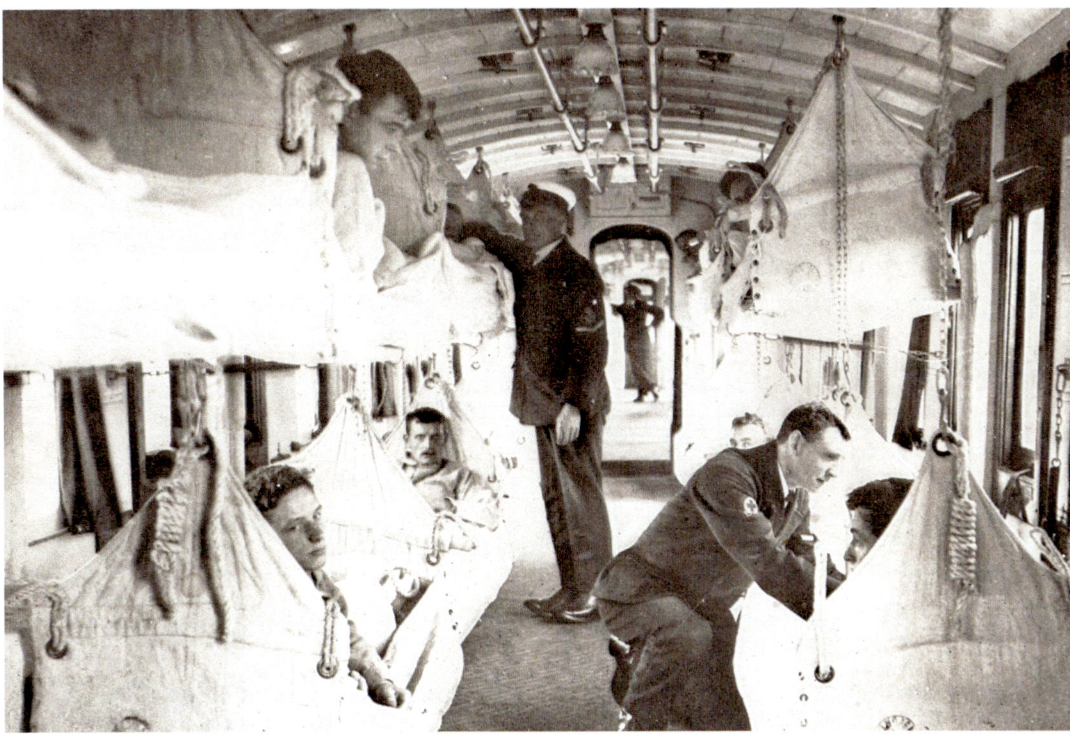

The interior of an RN (Home) Ambulance Train.

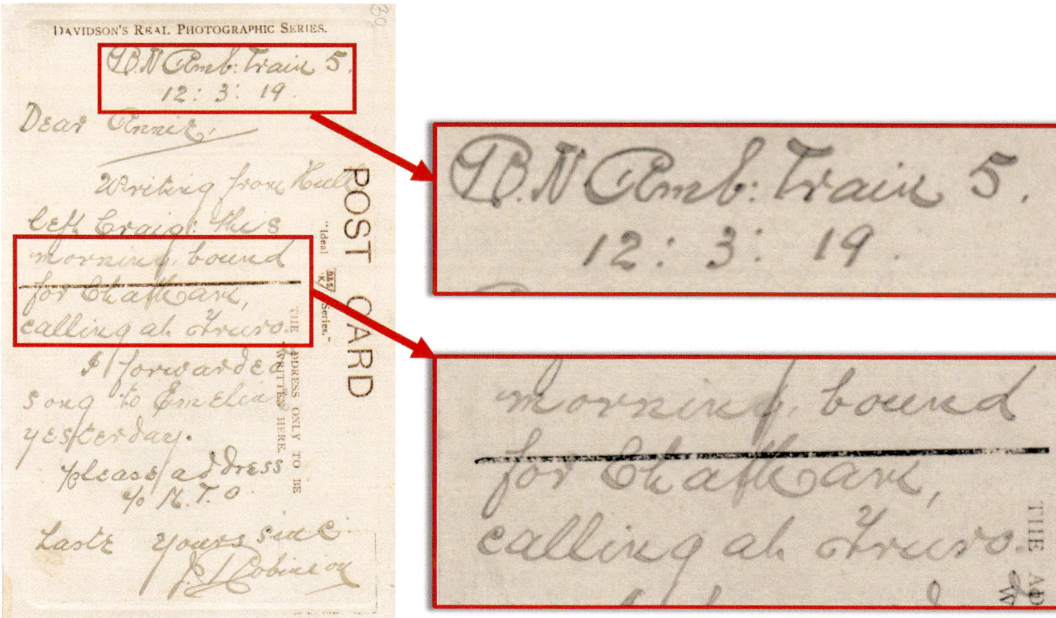

A postcard written from RN (Home) Ambulance Train No. 5 'bound for Chatham calling at Truro'.

the proceeds being donated to the Dreadnought Seaman's Hospital in Greenwich. Photographs were taken at the time from which postcards and stereoscope cards were produced for sale in order to increase fundraising.

Some of the east coast ports mentioned above were regularly used and continued to be so after the end of the war. A postcard survives written by a member of staff of RN Ambulance Train No. 5 on 12 March 1919. In the message the writer states: 'Writing from Hull ... bound for Chatham calling at Truro'. This rather strange routing included Truro as it was the location of a Royal Naval Convalescent Hospital that had been provisioned by the Cornwall Branch of the British Red Cross Society.[15]

It was considered that the Naval Medical Transport Service worked extremely well and Pratt states:

> In conjunction with the naval ambulance trains forming an essential part of the plan of operations, the Service, which worked with the greatest smoothness throughout, provided an elaborate and remarkable network of organised effort, and one that well deserves to rank among the most successful of British endeavours during the course of the war.[16]

HOME AMBULANCE TRAINS IN IRELAND

An aspect of the ambulance train story where records are sparse is in relation to Ireland. In May 1913 the War Office in London supplied the Irish railways with drawings of the LNWR ambulance train conversion with the instructions that two ambulance trains were to be produced and staffed by the RAMC in Ireland. One major difference lies in the fact that Ireland has a different rail gauge to the rest of Great Britain. The Irish rail gauge is 1,600 mm, or 5 ft 3 ins, as opposed to the 4 ft 8½ ins standard gauge throughout the rest of Great Britain.

The two ambulance trains provided by the Irish railways carried the numbers 13 and 14. Train 13 was converted by the Great Western Railway (Ireland) at their workshops in Dundalk and No. 14 by the Great Southern & Western Company (Ireland) at their workshops in Ichincore.[17] It is far from clear how these numbers came to be allocated. There was no No. 13 Ambulance Train within the rest of the British home ambulance train fleet, although there was already a No. 14.

The No. 13 Ambulance Train entered service in September 1914 and consisted of nine vehicles and was some 475 ft in length. The train had all the expected elements of ward coaches, pharmacy and treatment space along with kitchen and staff accommodation. One unusual feature was that the locomotive carried Red Cross emblems on white plates affixed to the front lamp brackets. The train carried ninety-six lying patients and had a staff of two doctors, two nursing sisters and twenty-one others, eighteen of whom were RAMC personnel. The other three were a cook, a cook's orderly and a compounder.

The first casualty-carrying journeys of No. 13 Ambulance Train were on 27 October 1914 from Queenstown Port to Cork and Dublin. Queenstown was on the south coast of Ireland and changed its name to Cobh in 1920 with the formation of the Irish Free State.

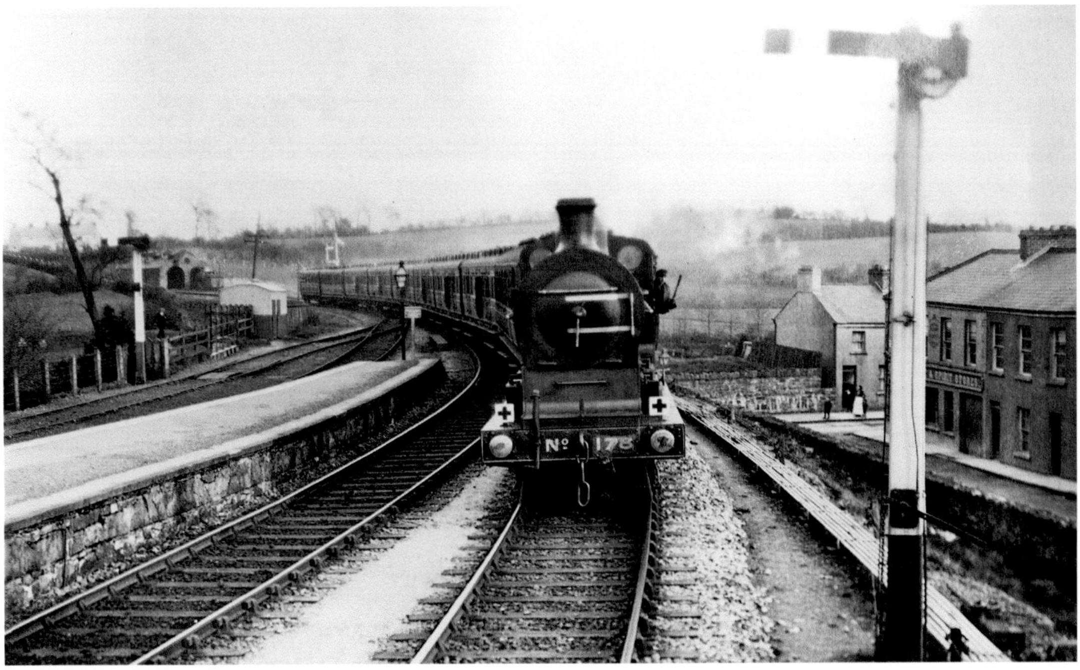

No. 13 Ambulance Train approaching Omagh on 1 May 1915. (Photograph by Norman Holland, courtesy of Alan Porter. Scan repair by Charles P. Friel)

Most of the train journeys collected patients from arriving hospital ships at Dublin Quays or Queenstown Port, Cork. Casualties were then distributed to hospitals across Ireland including Cork, Curragh, Belfast, Omagh and Derry although the picture is far from complete. The No. 13 Ambulance Train was decommissioned and the rolling stock returned to normal traffic in April 1919. The No. 14 Ambulance Train also started work on 27 October 1914 with journeys to Cork and Dublin and its rolling stock was also returned to normal use in April 1919.[18]

A long period of conflict in Ireland against British rule culminated in the Easter Rising of 1916 and the ensuing Irish War of Independence following, which resulted in Ireland being divided into Northern Ireland and the Republic of Ireland on 3 May 1921. This was to lead to a very different chapter in the ambulance train story by the time of the Second World War.

VOLUNTARY AID DETACHMENTS

The Voluntary Aid Detachment (VAD) system had been formed in 1909 on a county basis and by the summer of 1914 there were some 2,500 VADs across Great Britain. Although individuals were often referred to as VADs, the term actually meant a voluntary unit that provided nursing care, transport and other support to the military.

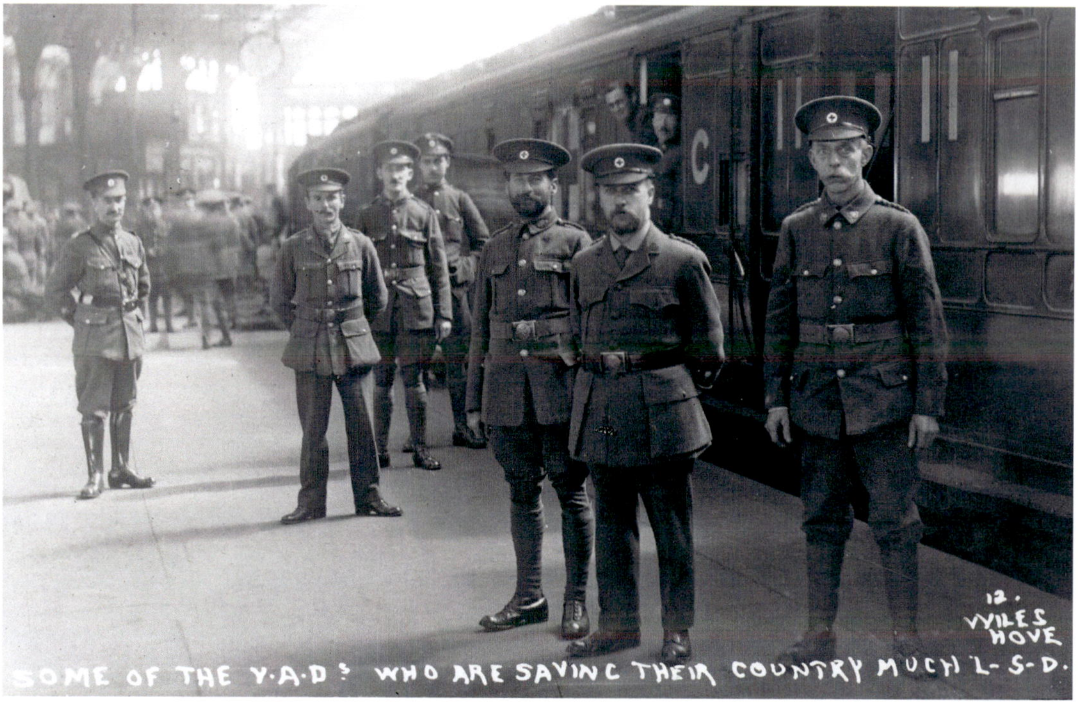

A postcard showing a VAD at Brighton Central Station supporting No. 11 (Home) Ambulance Train. (Garry George)

In October 1914 the Joint War Organisation of St John and the Red Cross was formed to better co-ordinate the work of the voluntary sector. The organisation consisted of the British Red Cross Society and the Order of St John of Jerusalem along with the St Andrew's Ambulance Association of Scotland. The aim was to avoid duplication of effort and to pool fundraising activities and resources. Everyone worked under the protective emblem of the Red Cross. Originally the VADs recruited both men and women, but as the war progressed many of the men enlisted into the army. Notwithstanding this, by 1918 there were over 80,000 VAD members.

The intended functions of the VADs were to be used in auxiliary hospitals, on ambulance trains, at railway rest stations, as stretcher bearers and for transport services.[19] Although service on ambulance trains is mentioned, it has not been possible to find examples of VAD staff working on ambulance trains during the First World War as opposed to what was to occur during the Second World War. VADs did however support ambulance trains at stations in stretcher bearer, welfare and transport roles.

Although largely outside the scope of this work it is fitting to mention that some VADs did go to France with War Office approval. The first to do so was in October 1914 when sixteen members from two London detachments established a Railway Rest Station at Boulogne. Here they fed wounded troops and provided minor care in support of the RAMC.[20] This was the beginning of a considerable network of rest stations and stores depots set up by the Joint War Organisation in France and Belgium in support of the military. The Joint War Organisation created for the First World War ceased operating in 1919.

THE FIRST OVERSEAS AMBULANCE TRAINS

On the outbreak of hostilities there were no ambulance trains readily available to be shipped to France, although plans were put in hand to convert stock that would be sent abroad. Therefore, the men required to operate ambulance trains were initially sent across with the rest of the British Expeditionary Force.

In 1922 Colonel G. A. Moore, writing under the pseudonym of 'Wagon-Lit', published a pamphlet entitled *The Birth and Early Days of our Ambulance Trains in France, August 1914*.[21] This publication was probably the earliest and undoubtedly one of the most important records of First World War ambulance train activity written by someone who was there. His first paragraph includes:

> …on August 4, 1914, six detachments, each of two officers and forty-five non-commissioned officers and men, Royal Army Medical Corps, and each designed for handling an ambulance train of 500-600 patients, found themselves camped on a hill-side in Aldershot…

A postcard survives showing the Redan Hill Camping Ground and the Government Sidings. This camp was no doubt the 'hillside' referred to by Colonel Moore in the

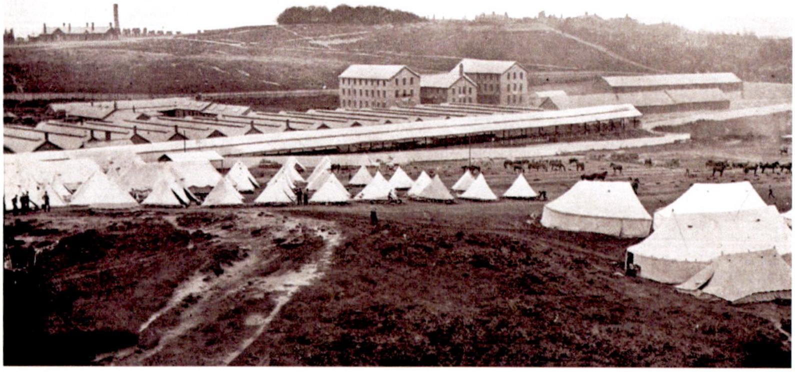

A postcard showing the Redan Hill Camping Ground and Government Sidings, Aldershot. The canopy running the length of the platform can be seen in the centre of the photograph.

above quote. His text continues: 'Early on August 13, the detachments entrained for a destination then unknown, and in the evening found themselves on the quay at Southampton. Next morning they were marching over the cobbled pavements of Boulogne. Two days later Amiens was reached…'[22]

Colonel G. A. Moore reported that it was at Amiens on 14 August 1914 that orders were received to form a British Ambulance Train Service at speed.[23] Moore continues: 'Accordingly, on August 17th at a large junction a mile from Amiens, 100 merchandise wagons, with a few passenger coaches and luggage vans were handed over to us by the French. This was the beginning of the British Ambulance Train Service.'[24]

These items of rolling stock were formed into the first three or four trains but many more were received because over the succeeding three months eleven trains were commissioned and commenced service. The table below shows the French Railway providing the rolling stock for each of those early British ambulance trains.[25]

British Train Number	French Railway Stock	Date of Service Entry
1	Etat	24 August 1914
2	Etat and PLM	25 August 1914
3	Etat and PLM	26 August 1914
4	Nord	30 August 1914
5	Etat and PLM	16 September 1914
6	Nord	5 September 1914
7	Etat and PLM	20 September 1914
8	Etat and Nord	8 October 1914
9	Etat and PLM	31 October 1914
10	Etat	13 November 1914
11	Etat	15 December 1914

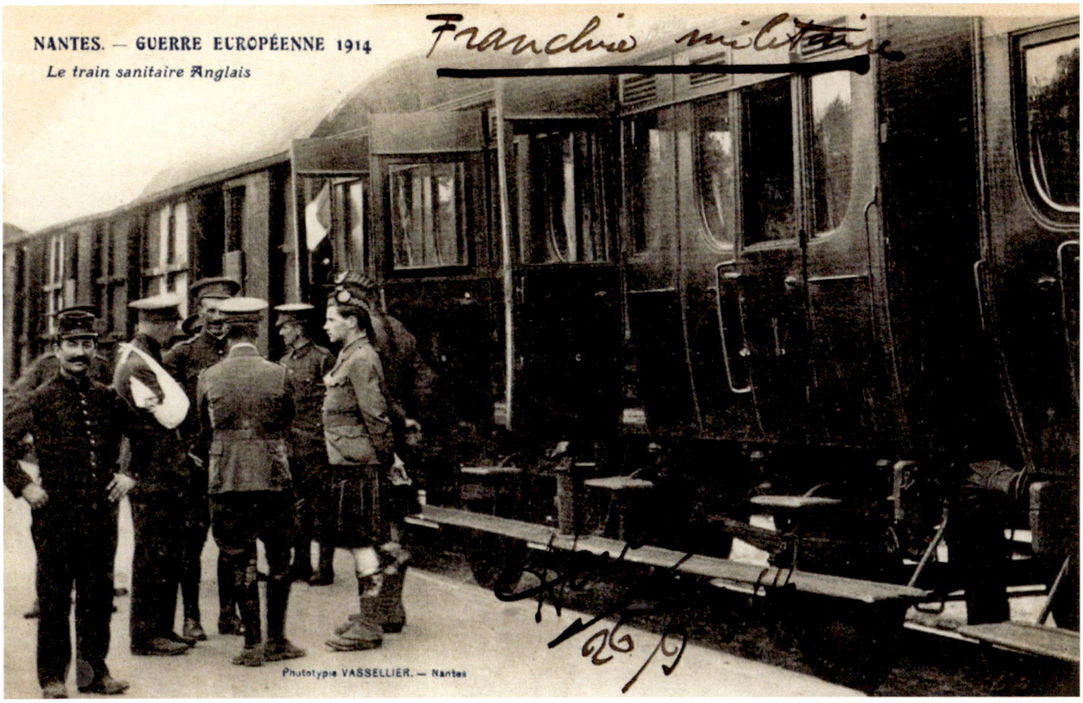
NANTES. — GUERRE EUROPÉENNE 1914
Le train sanitaire Anglais
Phototypie VASSELLIER. — Nantes

A postcard of an early British ambulance train consisting of French rolling stock at Nantes in September 1914.

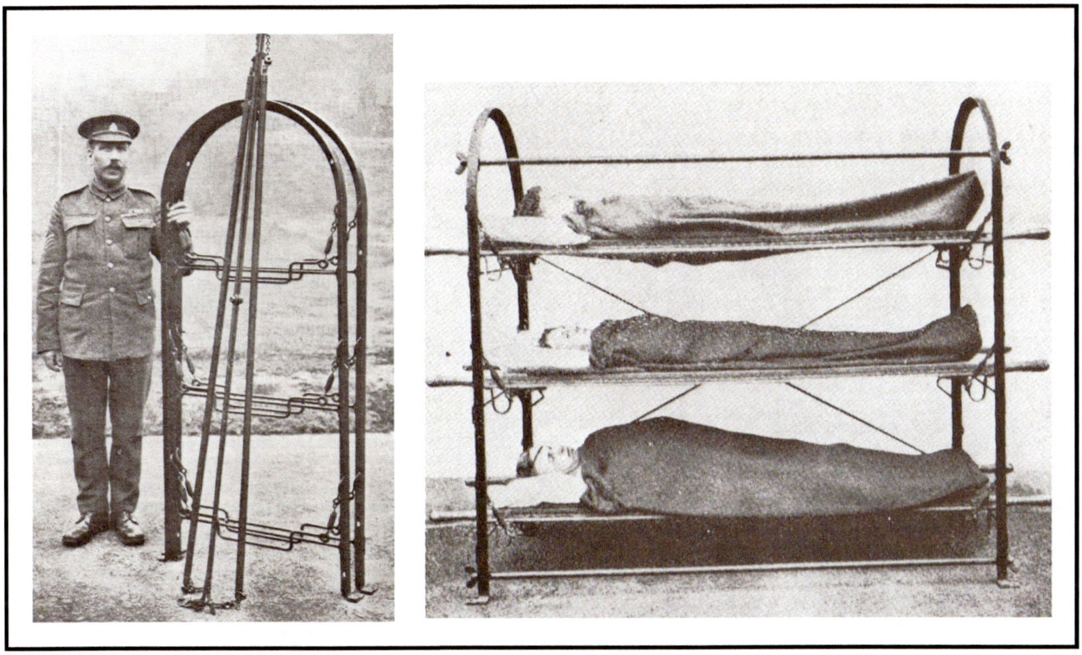

The *Bréchôt-Déspres-Amelines* (BDA) apparatus that collapsed for stowage and held three patients when in use.

In order to rapidly convert rolling stock to carry stretcher patients the British War Office had commissioned a supply of the *Béchôt-Déspres-Amelines* (BDA) apparatus to be sent to France. This was a collapsible iron structure that when assembled and fitted in any railway wagon would hold three stretcher patients.

The last of these trains made up from French rolling stock, No. 11, was funded and equipped by the British Red Cross Society and as will be mentioned in a later section was operated along with the No. 5 Ambulance Train by the Friends' Ambulance Unit of the Society of Friends, the Quakers, rather than the RAMC.

THE PROVISION OF AMBULANCE TRAINS FOR OVERSEAS SERVICE

When the shortcomings of the French rolling stock became apparent as well as the scale of increasing need, the first request for overseas ambulance trains came from the War Office in September 1914. Depending on the source consulted, these trains are sometimes referred to as 'Continental' with the abbreviation CAT, but the term 'overseas' with the abbreviation OAT will be used throughout this work.

From late 1914 the War Office created an Ambulance Train Committee which included membership from the British Railway Traffic Directorate, a British Army medical officer along with a representative of the French Military Railway Authority.[26] This committee's aim was to ensure co-ordination of the medical requirements emerging from France with the technical work required back in England to convert rolling stock for use overseas. From a railway operating standpoint various modifications were needed to couplings, draw hooks and steam pipe connections to allow continental running. In addition, American Westinghouse air brakes were also required which contrasted with the vacuum-braked HATs.

The Committee's work led to the evolution of a standard OAT that had sixteen carriages and was designed to take 320 lying and seventy-six sitting cases with forty-seven staff along with the train crew. The length of a train without the locomotive was 920 ft and weighted 440 tons. The individual coaches of a standard OAT all carried a designation letter that indicated their use and a train was typically made up as in the table below.[27]

Number	Function of Coach	Designation Letter
1	Brake van with a section for 18 isolation patients	S
1	Staff coach – officers	G
1	Kitchen and stores	A
4	Ward coaches with 36 lying patients each	B–E
1	Pharmacy and treatment coach	F
4	Ward coaches with 36 lying patients each	L–O

1	Sitting patients with a section for psychiatric patients	P
1	Kitchen	H
1	Staff coach – other ranks	R
1	Brake van and stores	T

The table that follows brings together details of the various railway companies converting rolling stock along with sponsors, where relevant, code names given to trains and the dates they entered service. This table has been compiled with information from a number of different sources.[28, 29, 30]

Train	Company Converting	Name / Sponsor	Codename	Exhibited	In Service Date
12	GER and LNWR		Paule	No	12 Nov. 1914
13	Number not issued			No	
14	LBSCR (9) and LNWR (7)	Queen Mary's Train		No	26 May 1915
15	Birmingham C&W Co	Princess Christian		No	1 Jun. 1915
16	GWR	UK Flour Millers		No	24 Apr. 1915
17	GER (15) and GWR (1)	UK Flour Millers		No	25 Apr. 1915
18	GWR		Carina	Yes	27 Sep. 1915
19	GWR		Yvonne	No	8 Feb. 1916
20	GER		Alice	Yes	5 Jan. 1916
21	LNWR			No	25 Aug. 1915
22	LNWR			Yes	20 Aug. 1915
23	Caledonian		Gertrude	Yes	3 Mar. 1916
24	LYR		Marthe	Yes	17 Sep. 1915
25	LBSCR		Suzanne	Yes	25 Mar. 1916
26	GWR		Elizabeth	Yes	14 May 1916
27	GWR		Arctic	Yes	24 Jun. 1916
28	GER		Adriatic	Yes	10 Jul. 1916
29	LYR		Pacific	Yes	26 Apr. 1916
30	LNWR			Yes	27 May 1916
31	LNWR		Jeanne	No	16 Jun. 1916
32	LNWR		Julienne	No	2 Sep. 1917
33	GWR		Gabrielle	No	28 Aug. 1917
34	MR			No	28 Sep. 1917

35	LSWR		Baltic	No	20 Dec. 1917
36	GER		Marie	No	12 Aug. 1917
37	NER			Yes	25 Nov. 1917
38	LNWR			No	21 Jul. 1917
39	GWR		Oceanic	No	28 Jan. 1918
40	MR			Yes	
41	LNWR		Madelon	No	12 Dec. 1917
42	LYR			Yes	16 Jan. 1918
43	GWR			Yes	3 Jun. 1918
44–51 were allocated to trains operating in other theatres of the war and converted overseas.					
52–70 were converted in British workshops and shipped to France for use by the US Army.					

Although the numbering is confusing, the table shows that a total of forty-nine OATs were converted utilising a total of 822 carriages and subsequently shipped to France.[31] The total appears not to include No. 40, which was later sent to Palestine, but does include the nineteen trains for use by the US Army that will be considered later.

Four of the earliest trains in the above table to be shipped to France were the result of philanthropy. The No. 14 OAT was donated by Lord and Lady Michelham and converted by the LBSCR. This train was handed over to the War Office at Victoria Station by the queen on 27 March 1915. It was subsequently known as Queen Mary's Ambulance Train after it entered service on 26 May 1915.[32]

The No. 15 OAT carried the same name as its predecessor from the South African War as it was sponsored by Princess Christian of Schleswig-Holstein. Also, like its predecessor, it was constructed at the Birmingham Railway Carriage and Wagon Company, which made it unique as all the other ambulance trains of the First World War were converted from existing rolling stock. Also, like its predecessor it was called the Princess Christian Hospital Train and was the only train in the First World War to continue to be called a hospital train. This title was carried on the sides of the coaches around the Red Cross emblem.[33]

Nos 16 and 17 (Overseas) Ambulance Trains were gifted to the British Red Cross Society by the UK Flour Millers Association and will be discussed more in a later section as they were operated by the Friends' Ambulance Unit of the Society of Friends, the Quakers, rather than the RAMC.

Each railway who converted rolling stock were proud to show off their contribution to the war effort. Companies recorded their efforts with photographs and brochures that showed their finished trains ready for deployment overseas. Commercial postcards were also produced for sale to the public. The public took great interest in the preparations being made for the care of casualties from the war and arrangements were made by several railway companies to tour their trains around their area of operations so that the public could visit.

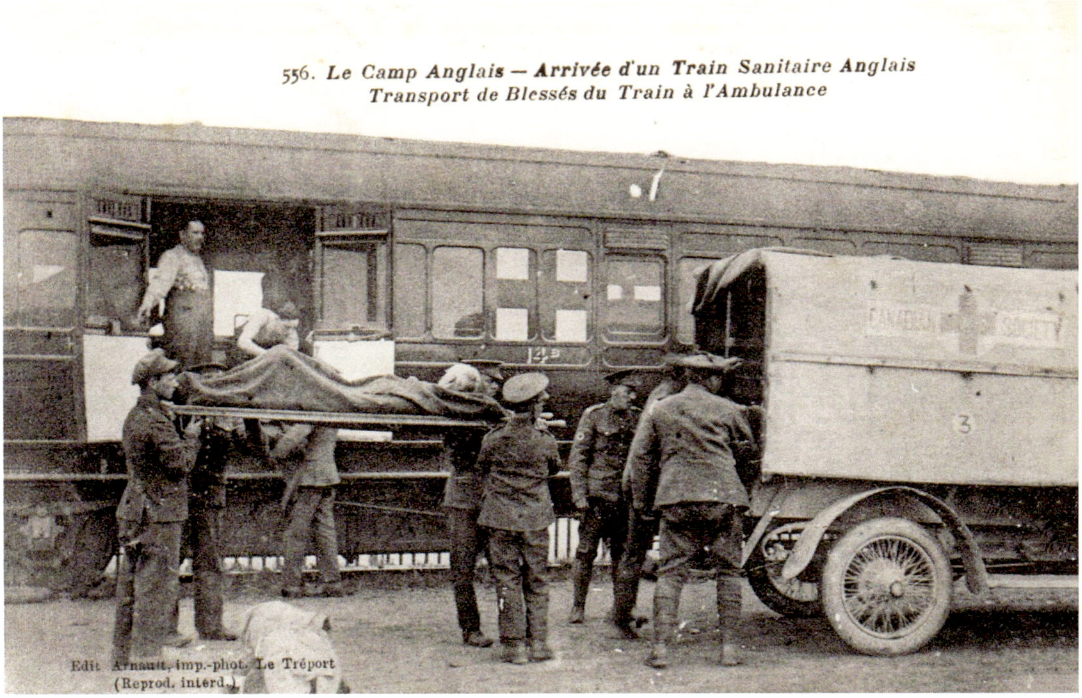
556. Le Camp Anglais — Arrivée d'un Train Sanitaire Anglais
Transport de Blessés du Train à l'Ambulance
Edit. Arnault, imp.-phot. Le Tréport
(Reprod. interd.)

A postcard showing a casualty being unloaded from No. 14 (Overseas) Ambulance Train into a Canadian Red Cross ambulance at Le Tréport in northern France.

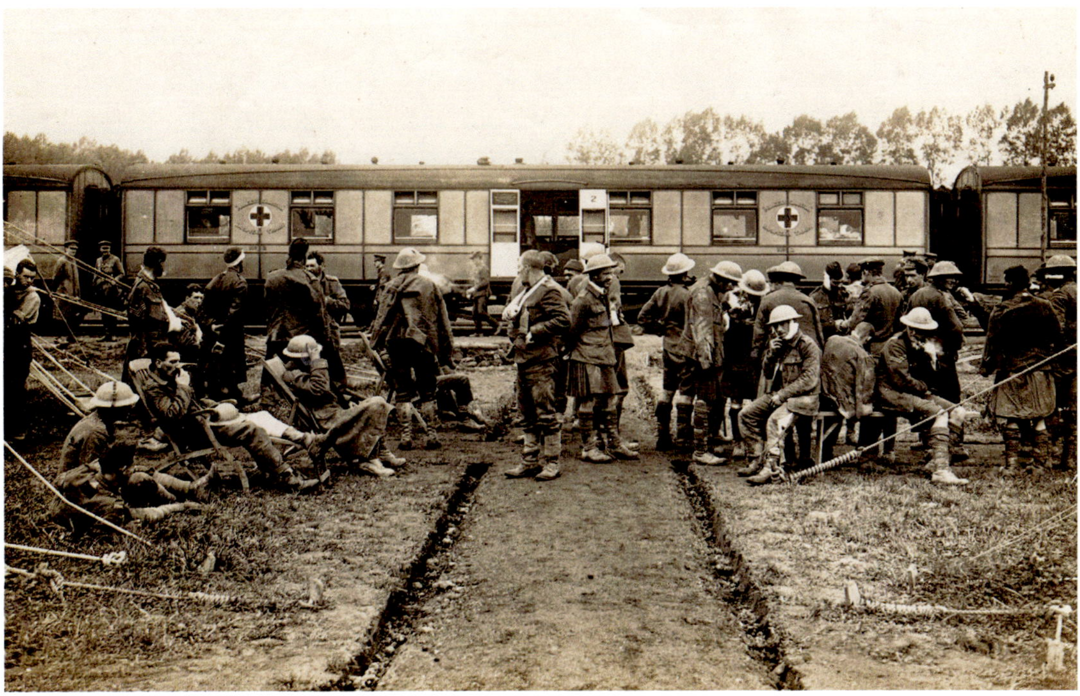

No. 15 (Overseas) Ambulance Train, also known as the Princess Christian Hospital Train.

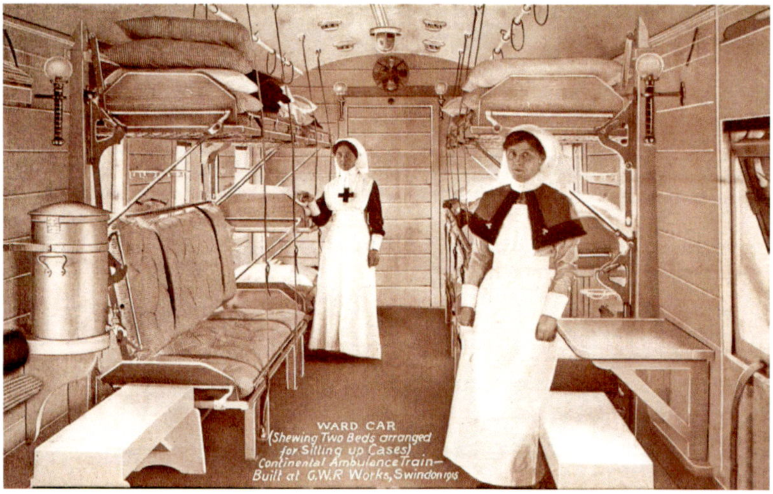

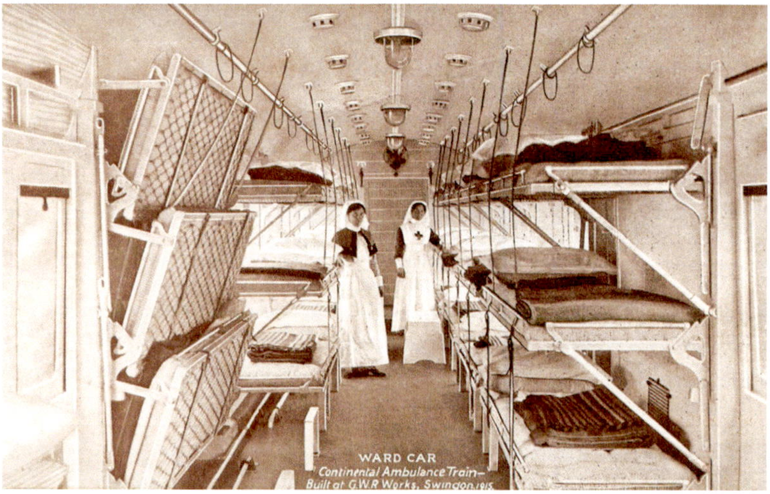

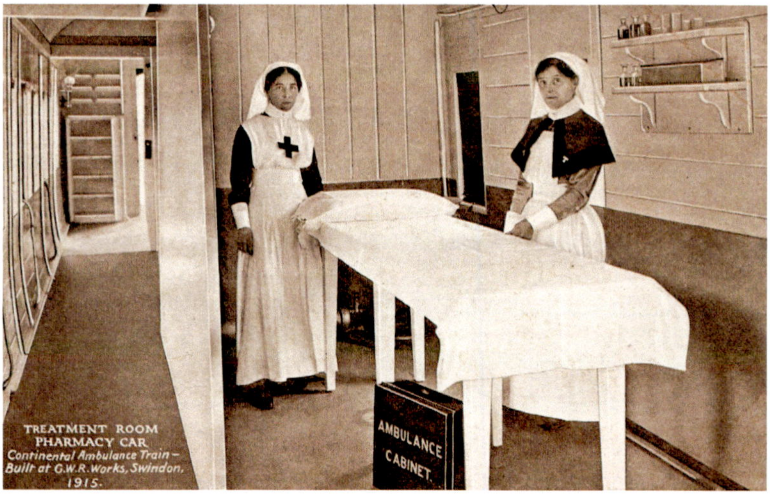

Three postcards from a set produced by the GWR to promote their ambulance trains.

No. 23 (Overseas) Ambulance Train was the only train to be converted by the Caledonian Railway and it was exhibited around the Caledonian Railway network. It was one of the standard OATs and was scheduled to visit Glasgow Central, Edinburgh Princes Street, Dundee West, Aberdeen, Stirling, Perth and Greenock Central stations. The popularity of the train lead to the addition of Motherwell, Paisley and a return visit to Glasgow Central being added to the tour. The admission charge at each station was 1*s*. (5p today) and monies raised were donated to the Scottish branches of the British Red Cross Society. It is recorded that some £13,255 was raised by over a quarter of a million people who visited the train.[34]

An official Caledonian Railway postcard of the train was also on sale and examples have been found of these cards posted at the various railway stations on the dates of the train's visits. One surviving example of this card was posted from Glasgow on 3 September 1915 and the writer states: 'You should see this train when it goes to Edinburgh. It is beautiful.'

Far more people visited the Caledonian Railway's ambulance train than any of the English railway companies' trains. Approximately a month earlier than the Caledonian Railway's ambulance train tour, the Great Eastern Railway promoted its sixteen-location tour of the No. 20 (Overseas) Ambulance Train between 5 and

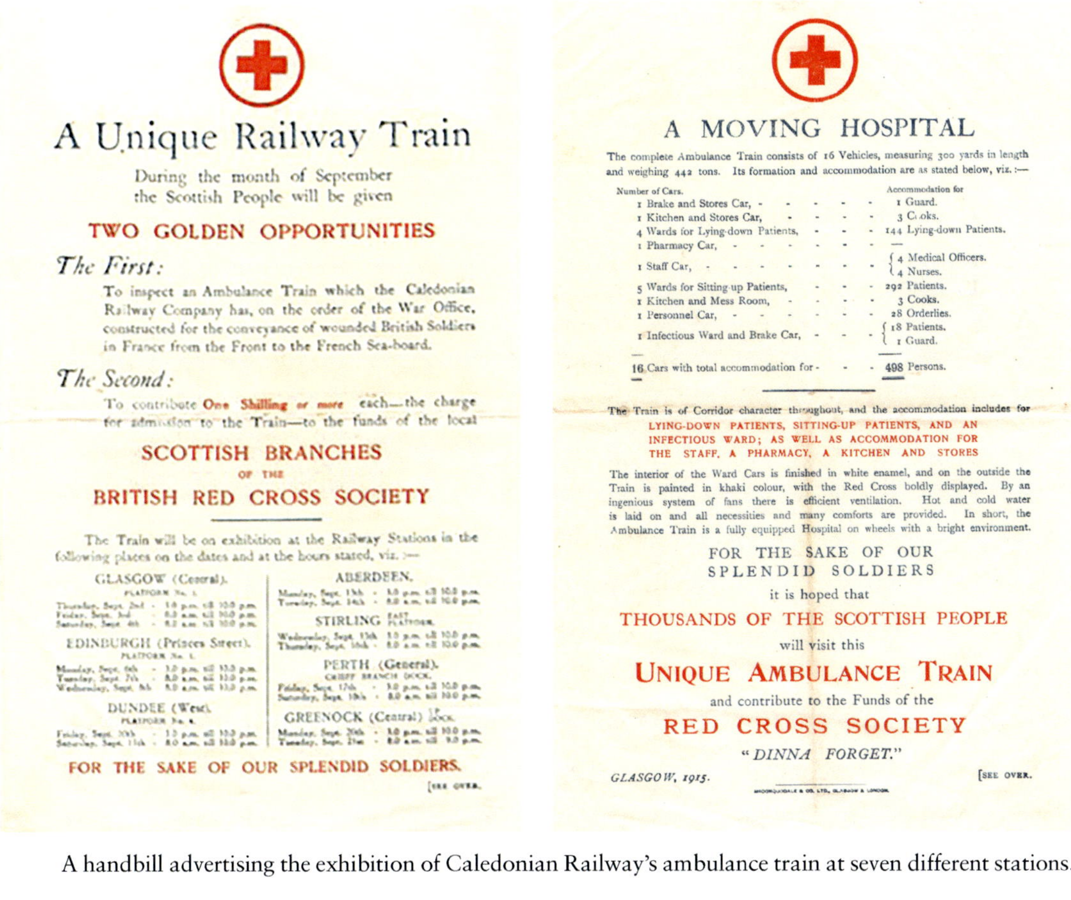

A Unique Railway Train

During the month of September the Scottish People will be given

TWO GOLDEN OPPORTUNITIES

The First:

To inspect an Ambulance Train which the Caledonian Railway Company has, on the order of the War Office, constructed for the conveyance of wounded British Soldiers in France from the Front to the French Sea-board.

The Second:

To contribute One Shilling or more each—the charge for admission to the Train—to the funds of the local

SCOTTISH BRANCHES OF THE BRITISH RED CROSS SOCIETY

The Train will be on exhibition at the Railway Stations in the following places on the dates and at the hours stated, viz.:—

GLASGOW (Central).

ABERDEEN.

STIRLING

EDINBURGH (Princes Street).

PERTH (General).

DUNDEE (West).

GREENOCK (Central)

FOR THE SAKE OF OUR SPLENDID SOLDIERS.

A MOVING HOSPITAL

The complete Ambulance Train consists of 16 Vehicles, measuring 300 yards in length and weighing 442 tons. Its formation and accommodation are as stated below, viz.:—

Number of Cars.	Accommodation for
1 Brake and Stores Car	1 Guard.
1 Kitchen and Stores Car	3 Cooks.
4 Wards for Lying-down Patients	144 Lying-down Patients.
1 Pharmacy Car	—
1 Staff Car	4 Medical Officers. 4 Nurses.
5 Wards for Sitting-up Patients	292 Patients.
1 Kitchen and Mess Room	3 Cooks.
1 Personnel Car	28 Orderlies.
1 Infectious Ward and Brake Car	18 Patients. 1 Guard.
16 Cars with total accommodation for	498 Persons.

The Train is of Corridor character throughout, and the accommodation includes for LYING-DOWN PATIENTS, SITTING-UP PATIENTS, AND AN INFECTIOUS WARD; AS WELL AS ACCOMMODATION FOR THE STAFF, A PHARMACY, A KITCHEN AND STORES

The interior of the Ward Cars is finished in white enamel, and on the outside the Train is painted in khaki colour, with the Red Cross boldly displayed. By an ingenious system of fans there is efficient ventilation. Hot and cold water is laid on and all necessities and many comforts are provided. In short, the Ambulance Train is a fully equipped Hospital on wheels with a bright environment.

FOR THE SAKE OF OUR SPLENDID SOLDIERS

it is hoped that

THOUSANDS OF THE SCOTTISH PEOPLE

will visit this

UNIQUE AMBULANCE TRAIN

and contribute to the Funds of the

RED CROSS SOCIETY

"DINNA FORGET."

GLASGOW, 1915. [SEE OVER.

A handbill advertising the exhibition of Caledonian Railway's ambulance train at seven different stations.

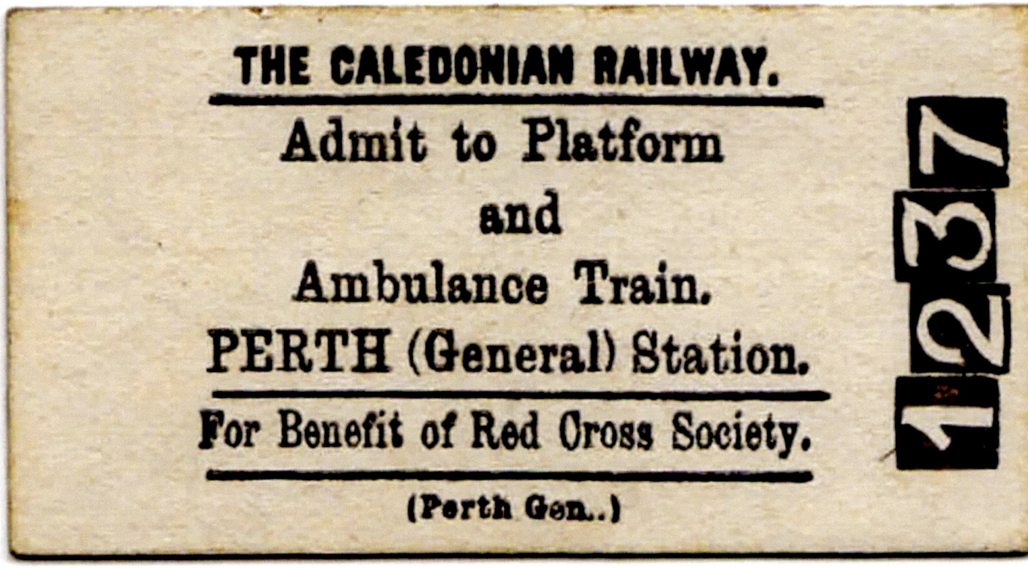

A very rare surviving platform ticket allowing public access to an ambulance train at Perth Station in 1915. (The late David G. Geldard, former editor of *Journal of the Transport Ticket Society*)

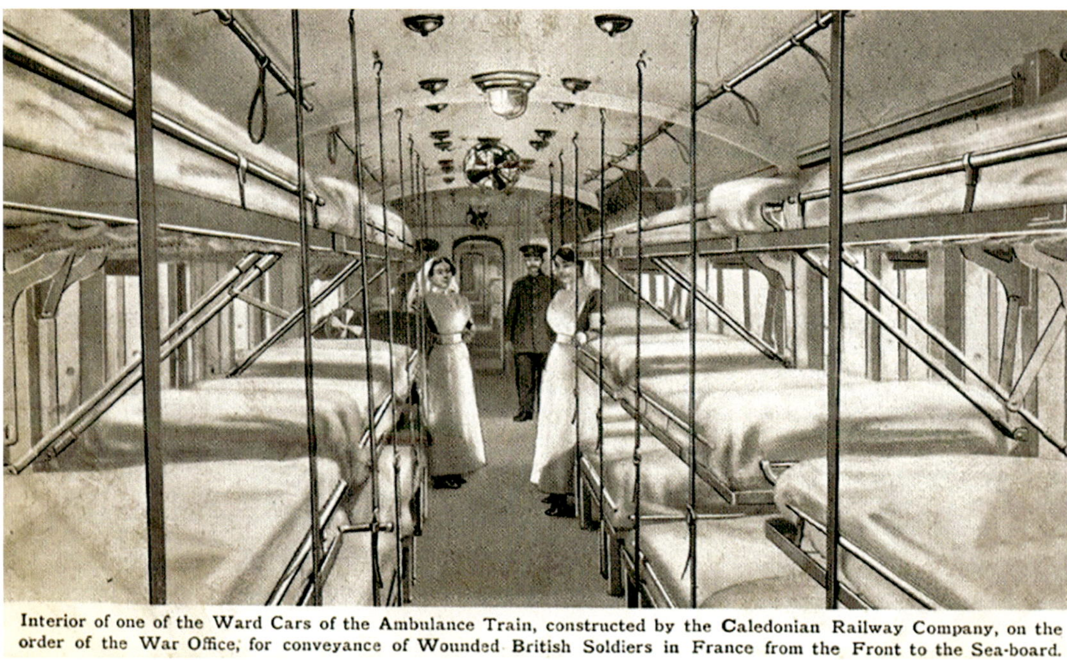

A postcard showing the interior of No. 23 (Overseas) Ambulance Train converted by the Caledonian Railway.

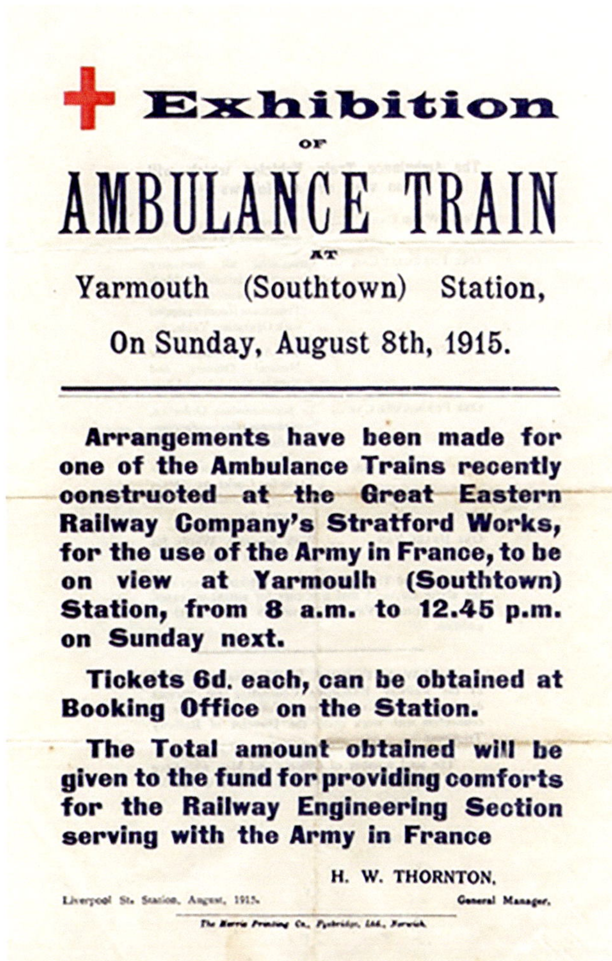

Exhibition

OF

AMBULANCE TRAIN

AT

Yarmouth (Southtown) Station,

On Sunday, August 8th, 1915.

Arrangements have been made for one of the Ambulance Trains recently constructed at the Great Eastern Railway Company's Stratford Works, for the use of the Army in France, to be on view at Yarmoulh (Southtown) Station, from 8 a.m. to 12.45 p.m. on Sunday next.

Tickets 6d. each, can be obtained at Booking Office on the Station.

The Total amount obtained will be given to the fund for providing comforts for the Railway Engineering Section serving with the Army in France

H. W. THORNTON,

Liverpool St. Station, August, 1915. General Manager.

A handbill advertising the exhibition of a Great Eastern Railway ambulance train at Yarmouth (Southtown) Station on 8 August 1915.

16 August 1915. One handbill from this tour invites the public to view the train at Yarmouth (Southtown) Station on 8 August 1915. Two differences here were that admission charge was only *6d*. (equivalent to 2½p today) and that all the proceeds from this and the tours by other railway companies' trains were being donated to the Comfort Fund for Royal Engineer Railway Troops serving in France.

During the early years of the war the prepared ambulance trains were shipped to France as freight with individual carriages being loaded onto ships by crane. This was not without its difficulties as very few ports had cranes capable of safely lifting carriages that weighed between 28 and 30 tons and had an average length of 57 ft. Dover, Portsmouth, London and Tilbury all had appropriate cranes, but in some locations additional railway sidings needed to be laid.

In view of the complexity of the task it is a tribute to the railway, dock and maritime personnel that records show only four out of the 822 bogie railway carriages transported to France failed to reach their destination in a usable condition.[35]

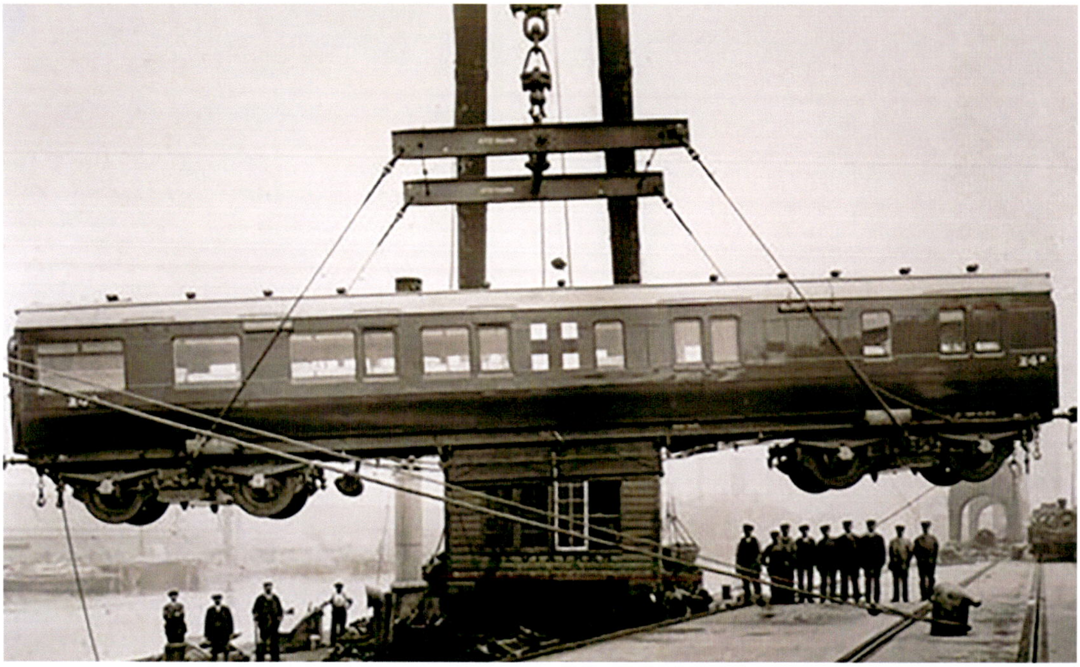

Coach B of No. 24 (Overseas) Ambulance Train being loaded at Tilbury Docks. (© The Board of Trustees of the Science Museum, Ref: HOR F1750)

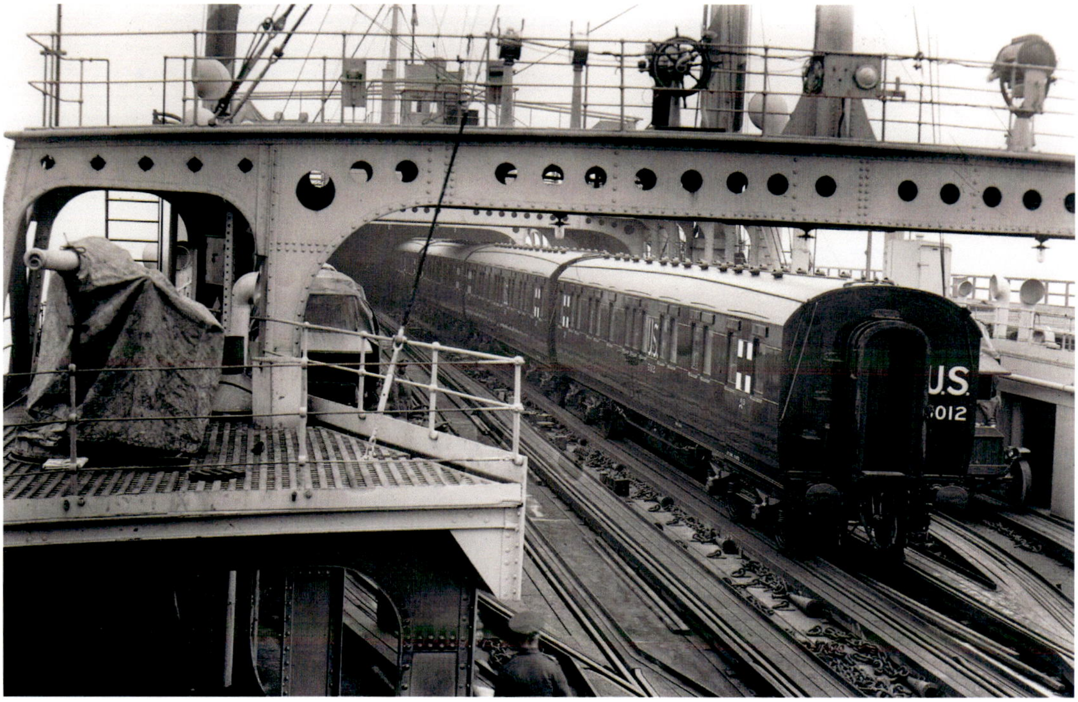

No. 60 (US) Ambulance Train on one of the three train ferries that operated to and from France. (© The Board of Trustees of the Science Museum, Ref: HOR F2531)

As the war progressed train ferries became a more efficient means of transporting the wide range of goods wagons, along with ambulance train rolling stock across the Channel. Three specifically designed train ferries were commissioned and a fourth purchased from Canada. *Train Ferry No. 1* and *No. 3* operated from Richborough Port, near Sandwich in Kent and *Train Ferry No. 2* from Southampton. The French Ports of Calais, Dieppe and Dunkirk were all used at various stages during the war. *Train Ferry No. 4* operated Southampton to Cherbourg.[36] The trains that were converted for use by the US Army after they entered the war were all transported to France by train ferries from Southampton to Dieppe or Cherbourg.

THE CASUALTY EVACUATION CHAIN – 'THE ROUTE BACK TO BLIGHTY'

The process of returning wounded soldiers home is often referred to as the chain of evacuation. During the First World War many photographs were clearly posed with smiles on all the faces of both patients and staff with the clear intention of reassuring the public back home that wounded servicemen were being well looked after on that long journey home.

The term 'Blighty' was an informal term used by troops during the First World War to describe Great Britain. Its origin is unclear and it could either be derived from the Hindi *bilaik*, meaning a foreign place, or the Arabic *beladi*, meaning a foreign country.[37] 'Blighty' became incorporated into military slang as a 'Blighty

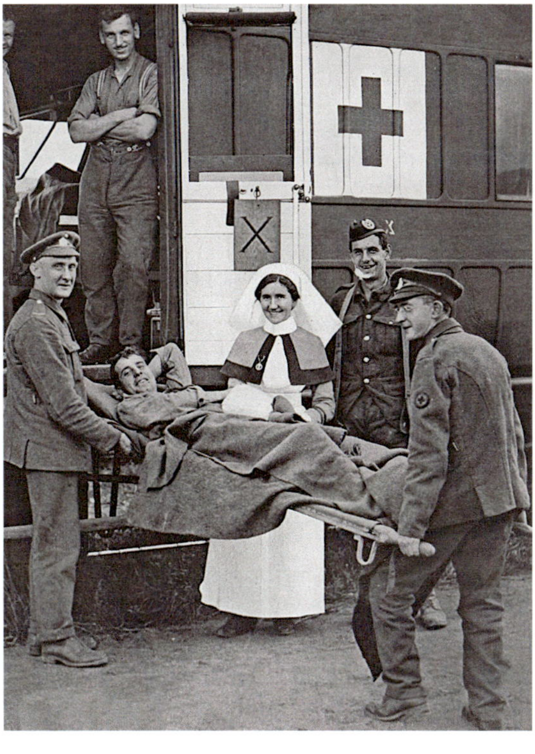

A posed photograph showing a patient being loaded into an ambulance train. The smiles were intended to reassure the public back home. (Alamy)

one' to denote a wound serious enough to ensure evacuation back home. Within the 'Route to Blighty', rail transportation was of major importance at every stage and was eloquently described in a memoir of an RAMC orderly's experiences at the 3rd London General Hospital in Wandsworth.[38] He details the arrival of casualties at his hospital by describing the arriving soldier in the following terms:

> Poor soul! – he is weary of 'giving his particulars'. He has had to give them half-a dozen times, perhaps more, since he left the front. At the field dressing station they wanted his particulars, at the clearing station, on the train, at the base hospital, on another train, on the steamer, on the next train, and now in this English hospital. As he sits and comforts himself with cocoa a VAD hovers at his elbow intent on a printed sheet...

As indicated in the quote above, from point of wounding any casualty could expect to spend some part of their journey home on one or more British or French ambulance trains. From the point of wounding a casualty would pass through a Regimental Aid Post, an Advanced Dressing Station to a Main Dressing Station and subsequently a Casualty Clearing Station. Transport between these would be

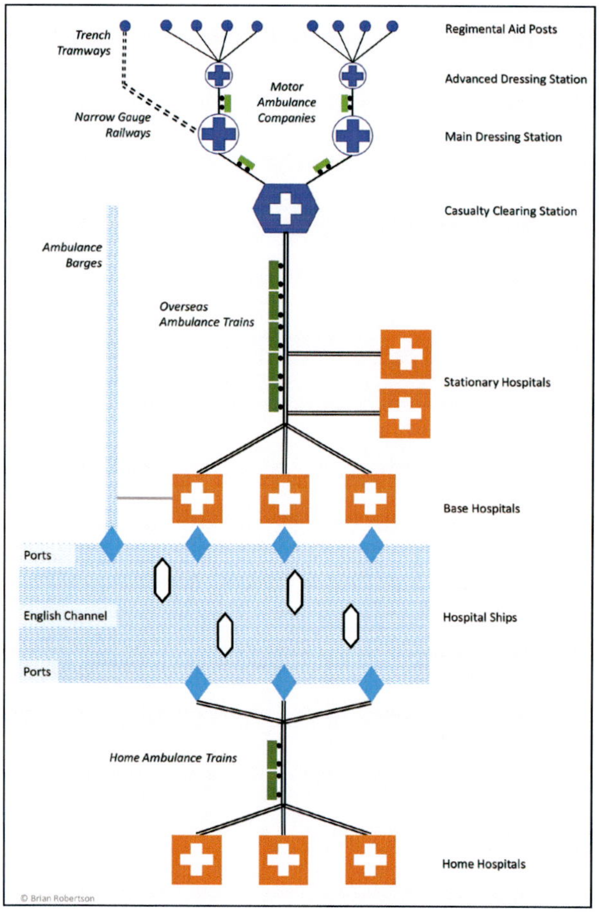

A schematic representation of the chain of evacuation for casualties from the front line back home to Blighty. (Drawn by Sally Finlayson)

by stretcher bearers or motor ambulances where available. There were also trench tramways and aerial ropeway systems within the trench networks. Narrow-gauge railways were also used in the forward areas to move casualties in addition to their more usual role of moving ammunition, stores and forage for the large number of horses. Narrow-gauge, patient-carrying vehicles were propelled by a mixture of man, horse or motor power. At any stage after treatment troops could be returned to the front unless they had suffered a 'a Blighty one' that would keep them moving along the evacuation route towards home.

A rarely mentioned element in the evacuation chain were the ambulance barges that were utilised on the canals and waterways of France and Belgium.[39] Early in 1915 four barges were funded by the British Water Ambulance Fund and were converted to take fifty beds each. Experienced canal barge operators were brought out from England to crew along with Royal Engineer soldiers. Each barge was staffed by a medical officer, two QAIMNS nursing officers, eight RAMC staff and three Inland Water Transport crew. Further barges were standardised at 126 ft in length with a beam of 16 ft 7 ins and carried thirty patients. The barges conveyed patients from forward areas to disembarkation points such as Amiens, Abbeville, Rouen, Le Havre and Calais, the first three of which were also major railheads. Only travelling in daylight, with a steam tug pulling one or a pair of barges the operating speed was just 3 miles per hour and by way of example the journey from St Omer to Calais took some eleven hours. Between 1915 and 1918 it is recorded that 70,059 patients were transported in ambulance barges as part of their journey home.

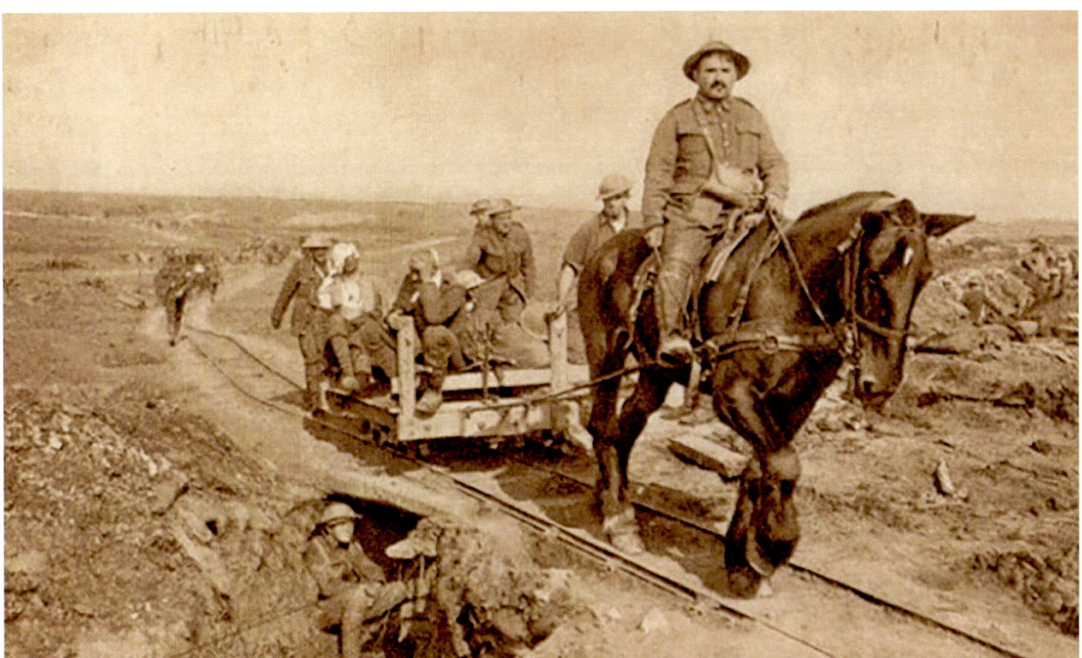

A postcard showing a horse-drawn, casualty-carrying, narrow-gauge trolley in the Canadian Sector of the Western Front.

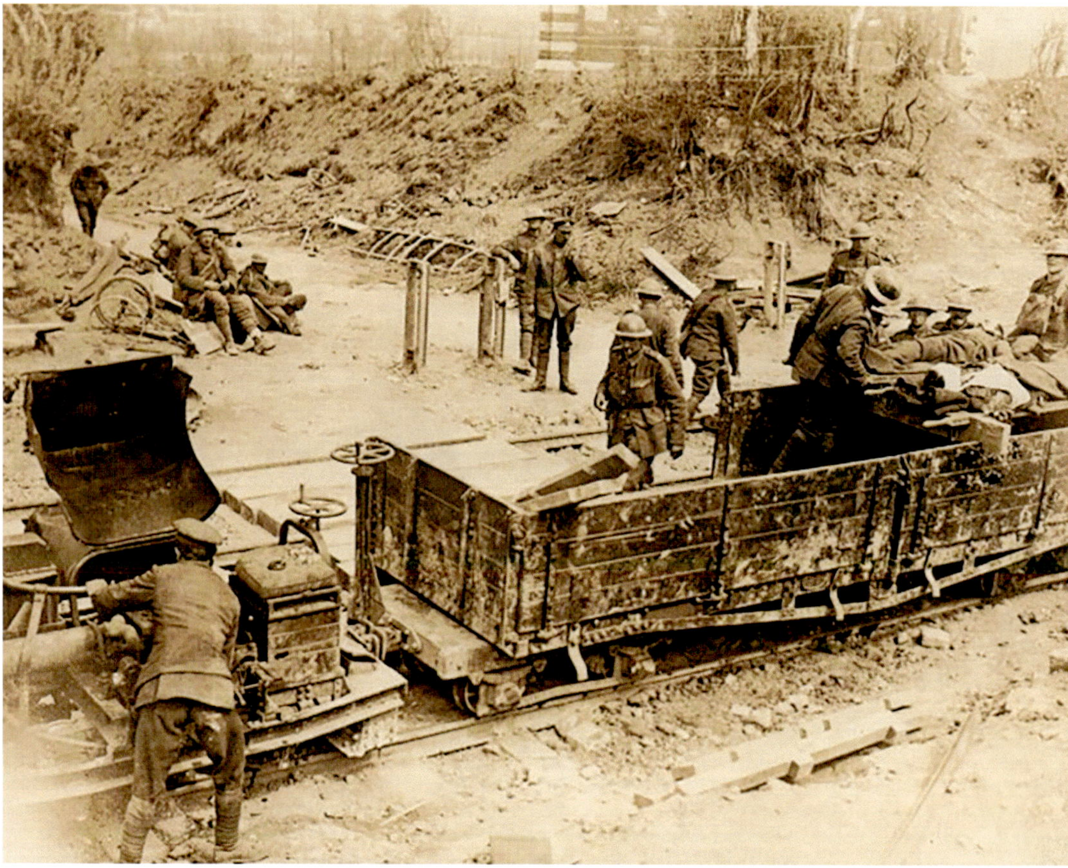

A narrow-gauge trench railway carrying wounded at Arras in 1917.

An interesting insight into the working of these barges can be found in some censored correspondence from a nursing sister who worked on them during 1917 and 1918.[40] On 13 September 1917 it records: 'I went into town in the afternoon and waded ankle-deep in mud most of the time so was glad to get back to my floating home.' By contrast on 3 May 1918: 'This has been a beautiful May Day – bright and sunny, with a light breeze. We half expected to load up today, but no other barges have come down, so we've had a very lazy day, most of which we have spent up on top, reading, writing and sewing.'

Ambulance trains were to be used to evacuate rearwards from Casualty Clearing Stations back to Stationary and Base Hospitals along with the Channel Ports. On the home side of the English Channel the casualties would be transferred to hospitals all round the country once again by ambulance trains.

The casualty evacuation chain along which the wounded soldier travelled on his way home is illustrated on a surviving Army Form W3118. This was a parchment envelope that contained field medical documents and of significance had space to record the various evacuation units through which the casualty passed. At the bottom of the front of the envelope is recorded that the casualty was loaded on

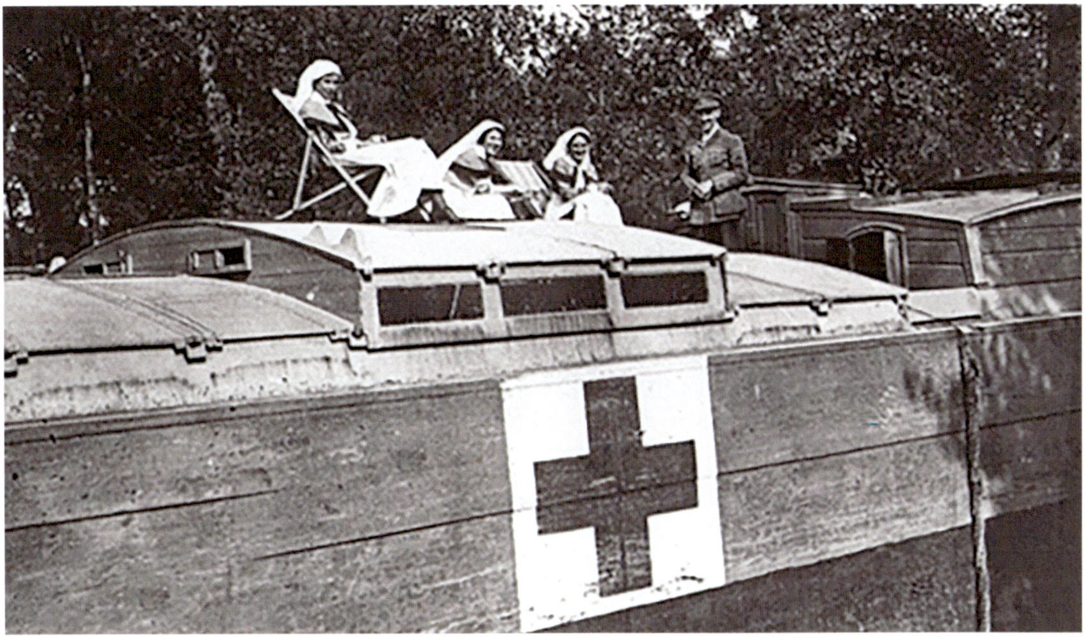

QAIMNS nursing sisters taking a break on an ambulance barge somewhere in France or Belgium.

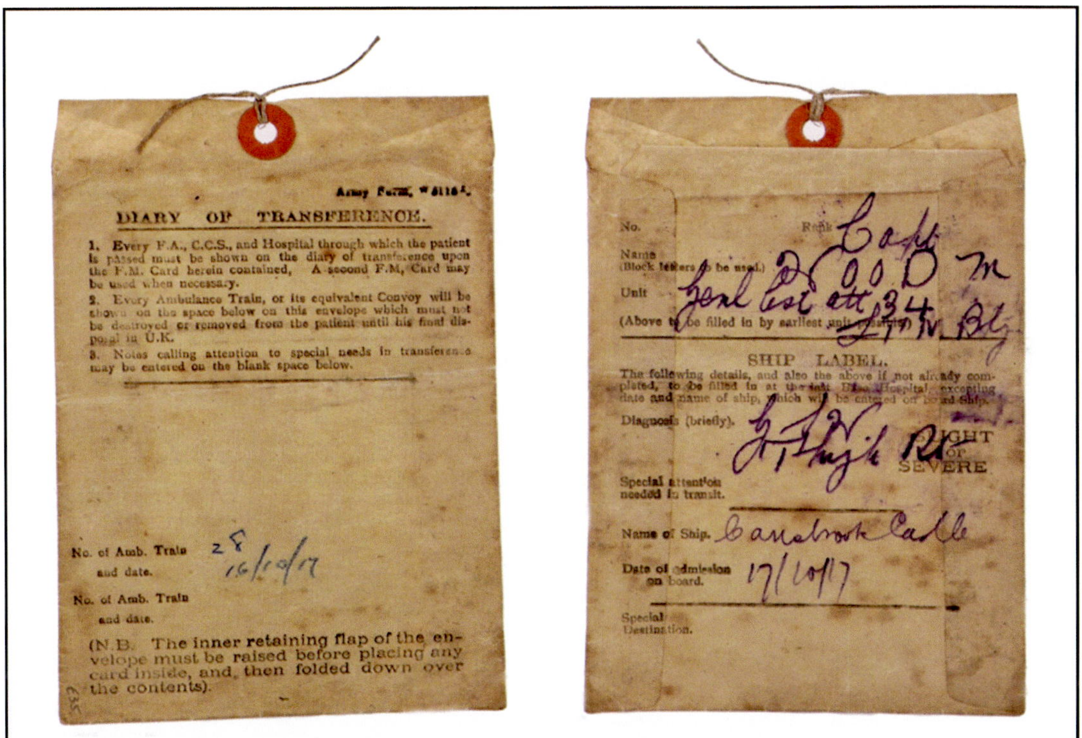

Army Form, W3118.

DIARY OF TRANSFERENCE.

1. Every F.A., C.C.S., and Hospital through which the patient is passed must be shown on the diary of transference upon the F.M. Card herein contained, A second F.M. Card may be used when necessary.

2. Every Ambulance Train, or its equivalent Convoy will be shown on the space below on this envelope which must not be destroyed or removed from the patient until his final disposal in U.K.

3. Notes calling attention to special needs in transference may be entered on the blank space below.

No. of Amb. Train and date. 28 16/10/17

No. of Amb. Train and date.

(N.B. The inner retaining flap of the envelope must be raised before placing any card inside, and, then folded down over the contents).

No. Rank

Name (Block letters to be used.)

Unit

(Above to be filled in by earliest unit possible)

SHIP LABEL.

The following details, and also the above if not already completed, to be filled in at the ... Hospital, excepting date and name of ship, which will be entered on board Ship.

Diagnosis (briefly). SLIGHT or SEVERE

Special attention needed in transit.

Name of Ship. Carisbrook Castle

Date of admission on board. 17/10/17

Special Destination.

An Army Form W3118 medical records envelope showing a wounded officer on No. 28 (Overseas) Ambulance Train on 16 October 1917.

to No. 28 (Overseas) Ambulance Train on 16 October 1917. Records show that No. 28 OAT was converted by the Great Eastern Railway and entered service on 10 July 1916.[41]

The reverse of the AF W3118 shows that the patient was an officer who had sustained a gunshot wound of his right thigh. At the bottom of this reverse side are details of the ship on which he was transferred to cross the English Channel. That ship was HMHS *Carisbrook Castle* which had been a Union-Castle Royal Mail Steamer built in Glasgow. It was converted to a hospital ship and served from 3 September 1914 until 26 August 1919 after which it was returned to Union-Castle Service until retirement in 1922. Its home port was Southampton. It carried 439 casualties and records show that in the month of October 1917 it did eight crossings to Southampton carrying 4,590 casualties of whom the individual named on the AF W3118 was one. Unfortunately, this AFW 3118 does not record the ambulance train to which he was undoubtedly transferred for his onward journey.

One high-profile journey along the casualty evacuation route followed an incident on 28 October 1915 that linked King George V with a hospital train, as described in the media at the time. The king had been in France visiting troops in Boulogne, Le Havre and Rouen amongst other locations. As he visited one group of troops, the horse he was riding was frightened by the cheering that greeted him, reared up, unseated the king and subsequently fell on him.

Despite the media reporting that the king was 'only bruised', the memoir of the Duke of Windsor stated that the king had suffered a fractured pelvis.[42] Some four days after the accident the king commenced his journey home in an ambulance train, although the details as to which one do not appear to have been recorded. What is recorded is that at Aire-sur-la-Lys, from his bed within the train, the king invested L/Sgt Oliver Brooks of the 3rd Battalion, Coldstream Guards, with the Victoria Cross for his actions at the Battle of Loos some weeks earlier.

Having travelled to the French coast, the king was embarked on HMHS *Anglia*, one of many steam ships requisitioned and converted for hospital ship duties. On 17 November 1915, only a few days after carrying the king across the Channel, HMHS *Anglia* hit a mine during a crossing to Dover. It was carrying 390 wounded servicemen and some 169 of the patients and crew sadly perished in the sinking.

OVERSEAS AMBULANCE TRAINS OPERATED BY THE FRIENDS' AMBULANCE UNIT

The Friends' Ambulance Unit (FAU) was founded by individual volunteer members of the British Religious Society of Friends, more commonly known at the Quakers. Known for their pacifism, this group of likeminded individuals set out to provide care facilities as soon as war broke out in 1914. They started life as the First Anglo-Belgian Ambulance Unit, but later changed their name to the Friends' Ambulance Unit. Their activities increased and they became responsible in part or completely for a number of hospitals both overseas and at home, a number of dressing stations in Belgium, motor ambulance companies, four hospital trains (Nos 5, 11, 16 and 17 OATs) and two hospital ships (HMHS *Western Australia* and *Glenart Castle*).[43] In addition, the FAU provided and staffed recreation rooms and canteens in Belgium and France where troops could relax, meet and socialise, write letters home, read newspapers and enjoy tea and cake.

With all the above development in the scope of the FAU, they were placed under the auspices of the Joint War Organisation of St John and the Red Cross but retained their own HQ in England along with a Continental HQ at Dunkirk.

With the passing of the Military Service Act in January 1916 and the subsequent conscription of all able-bodied men between the ages of eighteen and forty-one the FAU became an authorised alternative to conscription that allowed conscientious objectors to contribute to the war effort. It is often forgotten, however, that the FAU predated conscription and had been active for nearly two years by the time conscientious objectors were appearing in front of military service tribunals.

To concentrate on the FAU's contribution to ambulance train operations in France, the four trains for which they became wholly or partially responsible were taken over from other staff at differing times within the first two years of the war. No. 16 OAT was the first to be taken over in August 1915, followed by No. 17 in December 1915. No. 11 was next in January 1916, with No. 5 being taken over in August 1916.[44]

Nos 16 and 17 OATs were gifted to the British Red Cross Society by the United Kingdom Flour Millers Association. An appropriately inscribed doorplate was added to all the doors on the trains but only a very few survive.

Some interesting contemporaneous records from the FAU trains were published immediately after the war and draw on magazines produced by the staff whilst on

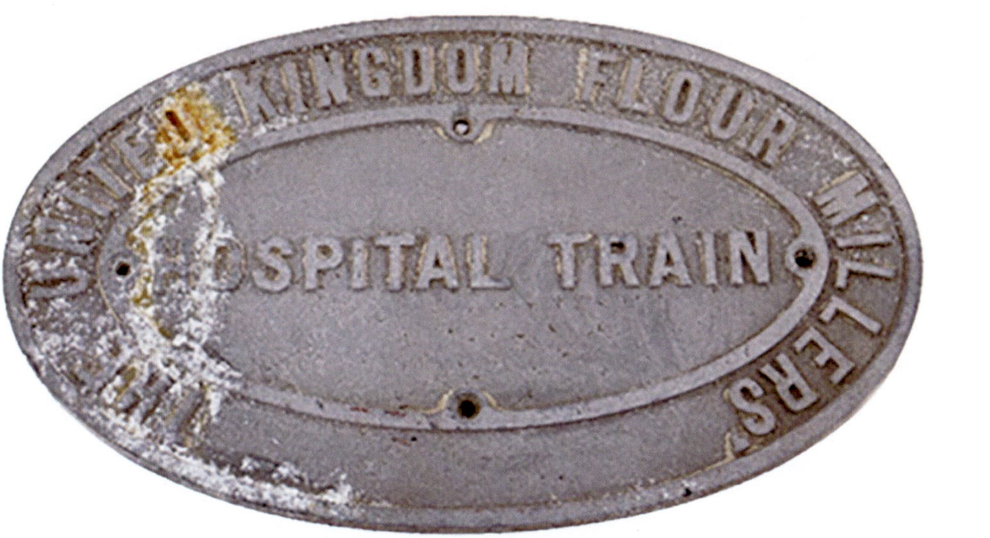

Door plate from the No. 16 or No. 17 (Overseas) Ambulance Train sponsored by the UK Flour Millers Association.

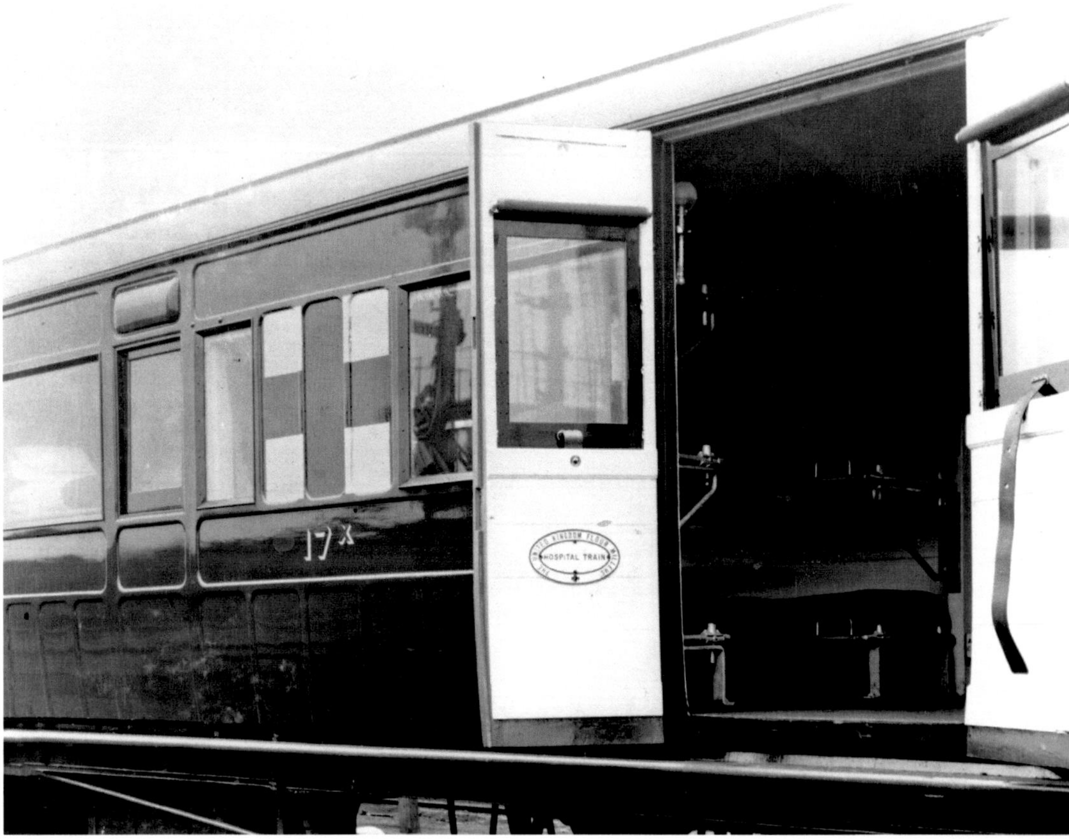

One of the door plates visible on No. 17 (Overseas) Ambulance Train. (© The Board of Trustees of the Science Museum, Ref: 1264/90)

active service.[45, 46] Both published in 1919, *A Train Errant* recounts details from No. 16 OAT whilst *Lines of Communications* was produced by No. 17 OAT. The production of magazines by ambulance train staff was also to be seen again during the Second World War and more recently during the Cold War.

No. 16 OAT was converted by the GWR at Swindon and consisted of fifteen double bogie coaches to which a French brake van was added once in France. It had a length of some 330 yards and a net weight of 460 tons.[47] A considerable amount of cleaning was part of train routine, and one of the staff wrote: 'It has been estimated that the white paint to be cleaned if extended in a wall six feet high would reach well over a mile. There were 708 windows to be cleaned and 800 blankets to be shaken.'[48]

Operationally, an insight into where trains operated was also given in that during the first year of the war trains operated two routings which they would work for a month at a time. The northern route evacuated casualties from the area around Poperinghe and Berguettes to Boulogne and Étaples. Trains operating further south of the front line evacuated patients to Rouen, Le Tréport, Etrétat and Le Havre.[49]

No. 17 OAT was converted by the GER at their Stratford works in East London to a similar specification as No. 16. Having been shipped across from England,

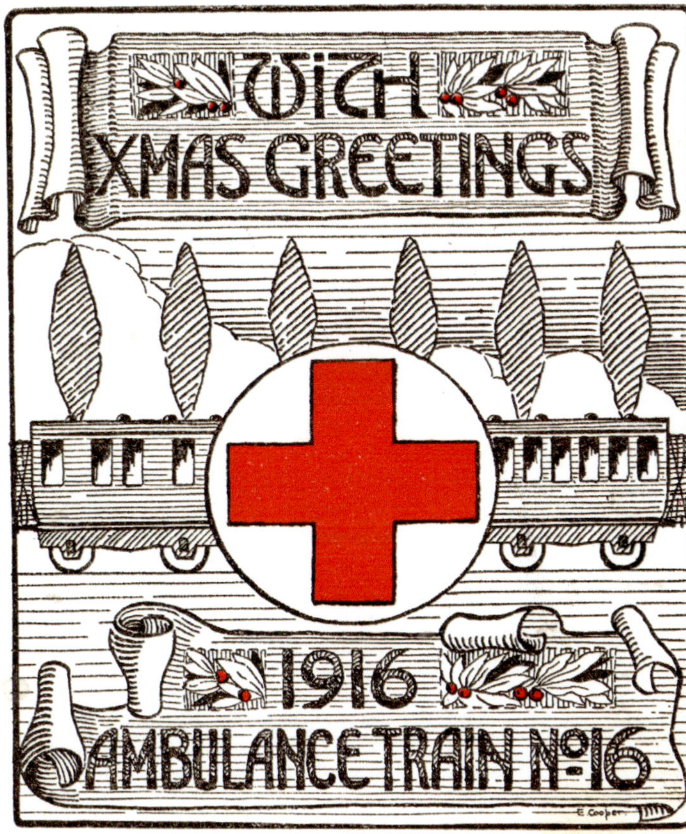

A 1916 Christmas card from a member of staff on No. 16 Ambulance Train in France. The original envelope that has survived is annotated 'On Active Service' and carries an 'ARMY PO 3' cancellation dated 18 December 1916. This APO is recorded as being at Boulogne.

initially two French brake vans were added but were replaced by GER vehicles. No. 17 Ambulance Train entered service on 25 April 1915 with an RAMC Staff. An RAMC embroidered silk postcard has survived and confirms this in that the sender datelines the card 'No 17 Ambulance Train BEF France'.

Records show that FAU personnel destined for this train crossed the Channel and arrived in Boulogne on 28 November 1915, but did not take over the No. 17 OAT rolling stock until 2 December 1915. There is an interesting comment concerning this in their souvenir publication, *Lines of Communication*:

> We left for France at the end of November, and after waiting a week at a base town for a train to come in, we joined just in time to see the previous personnel leave. Not till we got to France did we realise that we were to replace paid men already on the train.[50]

This publication is described on the frontispiece as 'being pages from the Train Magazines which were published whilst on Active Service, together with descriptions of Ambulance Train life'. Just as its fellow publication, *A Train Errant*, it contains a wealth of information concerning the train, its organisation and staff often missing from more formal histories. Of particular interest is a diary of the activities and

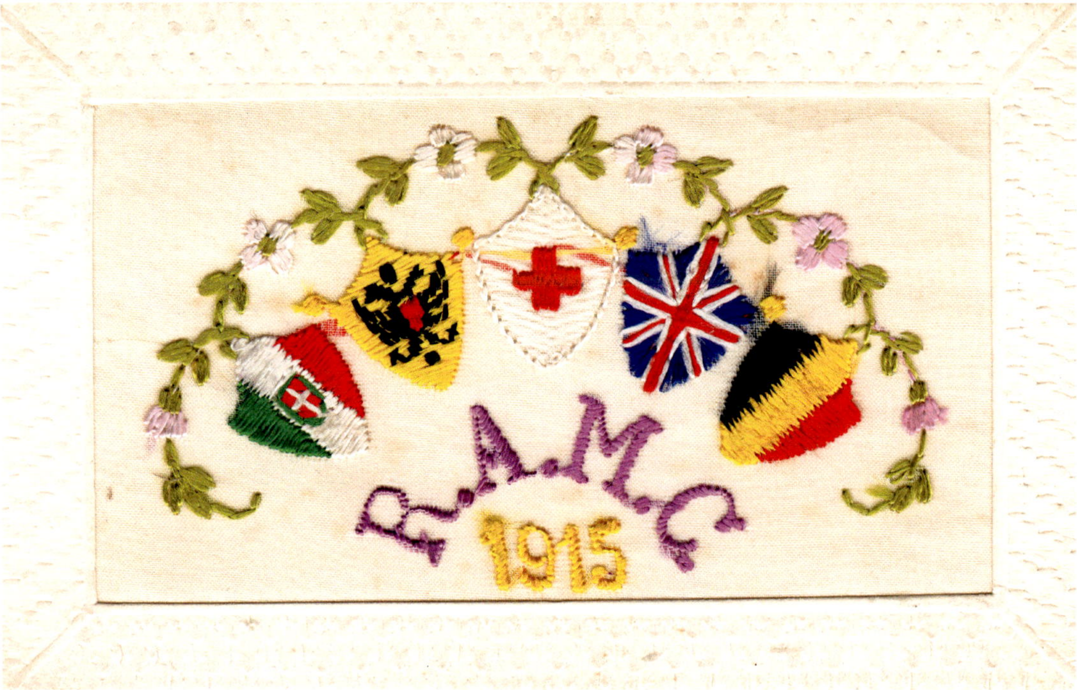

An embroidered silk postcard datelined 'No 17 Ambulance Train BEF France'.

movements of the train from 28 November 1915 until 2 February 1919. There are lists of the major engagements from which the train carried casualties as well as detailed tables of casualty statistics by day and month throughout the time the FAU was operating the train.

Some statistics illustrate the contribution made by the FAU personnel staffing this train to the overall casualty evacuation effort. The total number of trips before the FAU took over No. 17 OAT was sixty-six and after it was 376. The total number of patients carried before the FAU took over was 19,936 and during their operation of the train 136,616. The train was recorded as having covered approximately 62,782 miles.[51]

Mention must be made of the other two trains operated by the FAU. The FAU took over No. 11 in January 1916. This was one of the early British ambulance trains that consisted of rolling stock acquired from the French Etat railway. The last train to be taken over by the FAU was No. 5 in August 1916 and this, too, was French rolling stock from two different Companies Etat and PLM. Records show that staff were moved between the trains as required.

By the end of the war, having started with just forty FAU volunteers travelling to France, there were over 640 serving in France with another 720 active in the FAU's Home Service Section. After the Armistice the FAU continued to provide their services until their disbandment in 1919.[52]

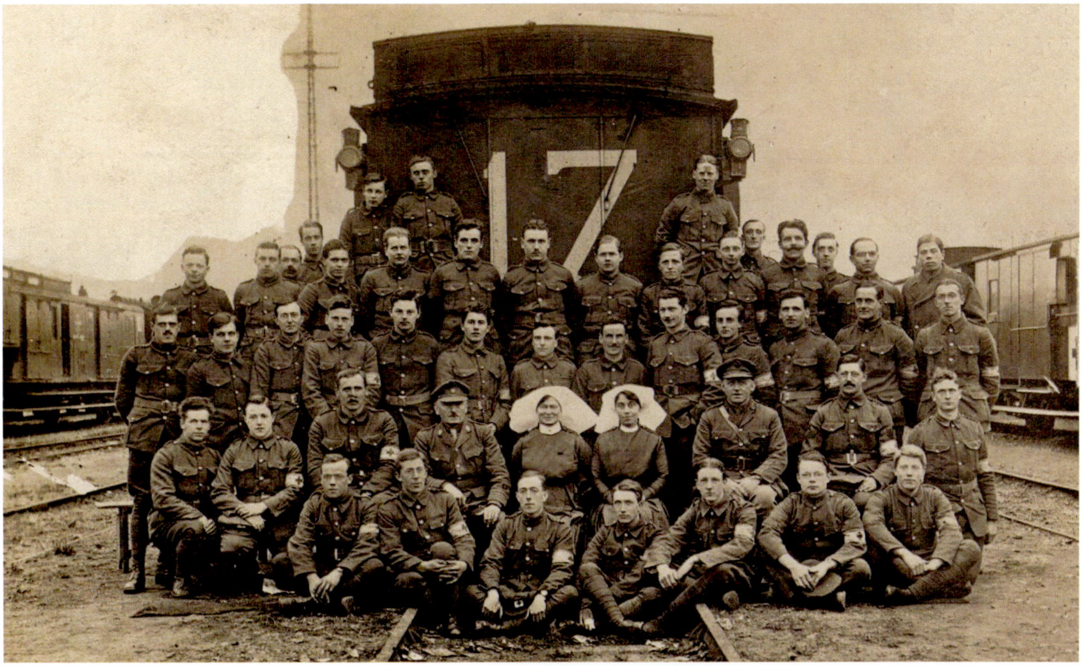

Above: Staff of No. 17 (Overseas) Ambulance Train somewhere in France.

Right: The interior of No. 17 (Overseas) Ambulance Train.

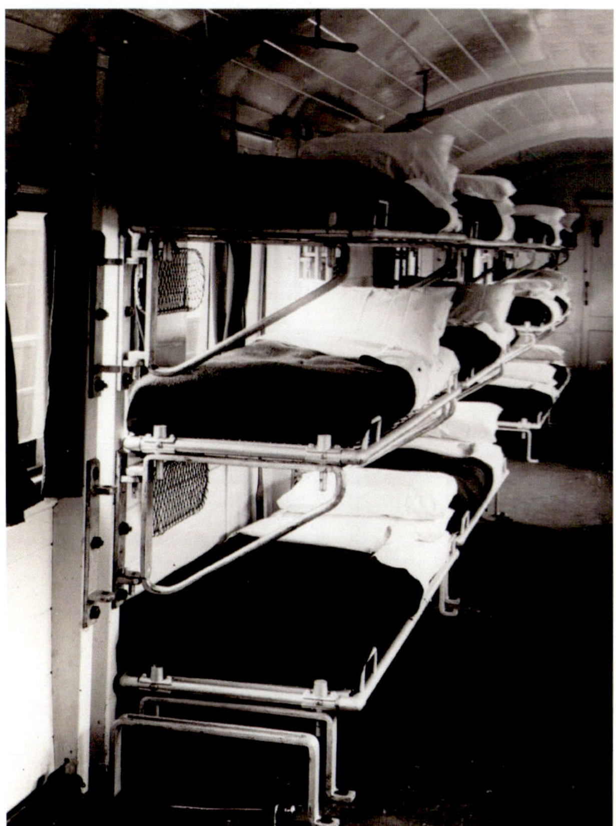

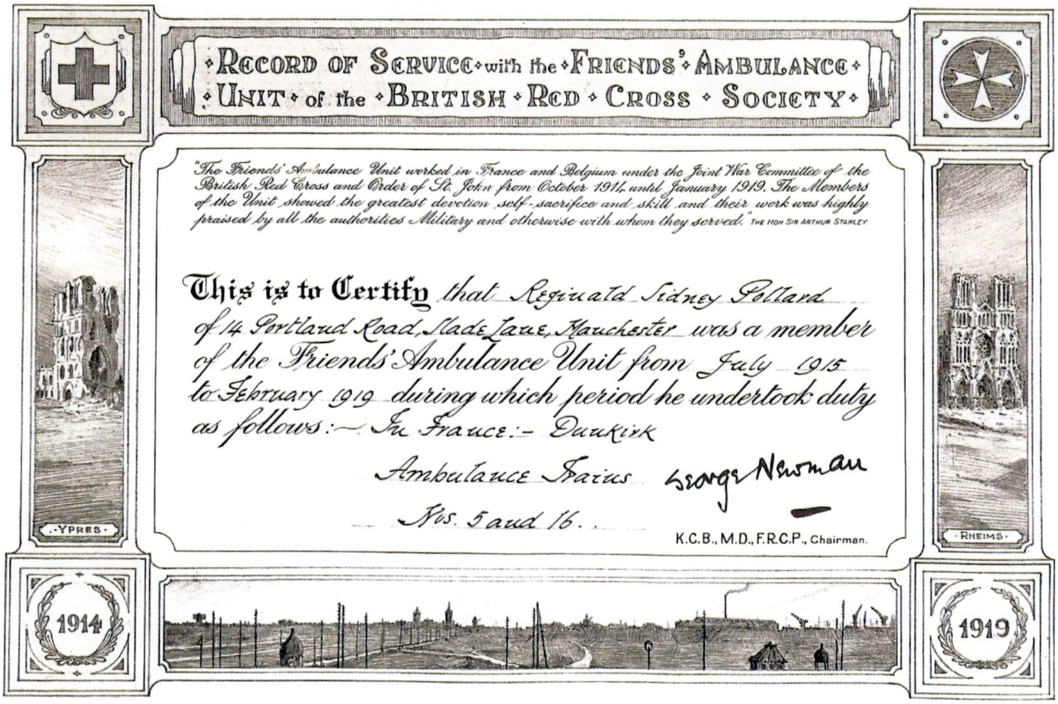

RECORD OF SERVICE with the FRIENDS' AMBULANCE UNIT of the BRITISH RED CROSS SOCIETY

"The Friends' Ambulance Unit worked in France and Belgium under the Joint War Committee of the British Red Cross and Order of St. John from October 1914 until January 1919. The Members of the Unit showed the greatest devotion, self-sacrifice and skill and their work was highly praised by all the authorities Military and otherwise with whom they served." THE HON SIR ARTHUR STANLEY

This is to Certify that Reginald Sidney Pollard of 14 Portland Road, Slade Lane, Manchester was a member of the Friends' Ambulance Unit from July 1915 to February 1919 during which period he undertook duty as follows:— In France:- Dunkirk Ambulance Trains Nos. 5 and 16.

George Newman
K.C.B., M.D., F.R.C.P., Chairman.

YPRES · RHEIMS · 1914 · 1919

A certificate of service awarded to a member of the FAU who served on Nos 5 and 16 Ambulance Trains. (British Red Cross Museum and Archives)

OVERSEAS AMBULANCE TRAINS OPERATED BY AMERICAN FORCES

The USA entered the First World War on 4 April 1917 and a decision was made that ambulance trains for use by American forces in France would be converted in England then shipped to France to await the arrival of American medical personnel with the American Expeditionary Force (AEF). The first order for ambulance trains for the Americans to use was placed in August 1917, and by the end of the war nineteen standard OATs consisting of some 304 bogie carriages had been delivered. Of these trains five were constructed by the Midland Railway, four each by GWR and LNWR, three by LRY and one each by GCR, GER and LSWR. A further twenty-nine ambulance trains to be operated by American forces were on order at the time the Armistice was eventually signed on 11 November 1918.[53]

The one train converted by the LSWR was designated No. 62 (US) Ambulance Train and consisted of fourteen corridor coaches each 56 ft in length along with two vans. Characteristically, each of the trains used by the Americans had their number and 'US' in large letters on the end and sides of the coaches. No. 62 was configured to carry 418 lying patients or 680 walking casualties.[54]

This LSWR train was put on display at London's Waterloo Station between 16 and 18 May 1918. Unlike many of the other sites where trains were open to

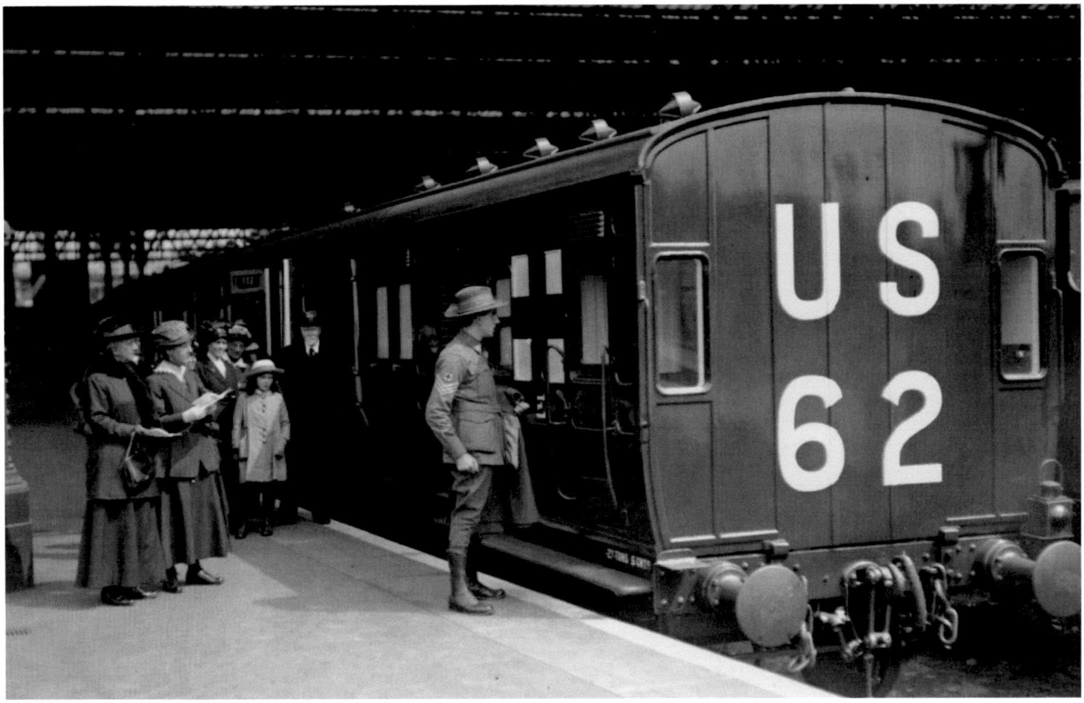

No. 62 (US) Ambulance Train on show to the public at Waterloo Station in London prior to deployment to France.

the public, the admission charge to this train was 8*d*. The funds collected were distributed between St Dunstan's Hostel for Blinded Soldiers and Sailors (now Blind Veterans UK), St John Ambulance and the South-Western Railway Servants' Orphanage Fund.[55] The public took great interest in these trains and four of the US trains were exhibited around the country.

An interesting insight into the operating of one of these American trains was found in a collection of documents, photographs, military forms and ephemera purchased at auction in June 2020. They all related to an American serviceman on No. 55 (US) Ambulance Train. One document was a historical report documenting the train's activities between 1 January 1918 and 1 January 1919. At this period American forces were still using the term 'hospital train' and this document describes hospital train No. 32 being organised at Fort Sheridan in Illinois in January 1918. On 10 May 1918 the unit sailed from Hoboken, New Jersey, as part of the AEF, arriving at Brest in France on 25 May 1918. They then moved by train to Corvol-d'Embernard where an ambulance train carrying the No. 55 was waiting. The unit had left America as hospital train No. 32, but British No. 32 (Overseas) Ambulance Train was already operating in Europe. Therefore, this American unit became and operated as No. 55 (US) Ambulance Train. This change of train number also occurred to other American-operated ambulance trains which undoubtedly fuelled some of the confusion surrounding ambulance train numbering during the First World War.

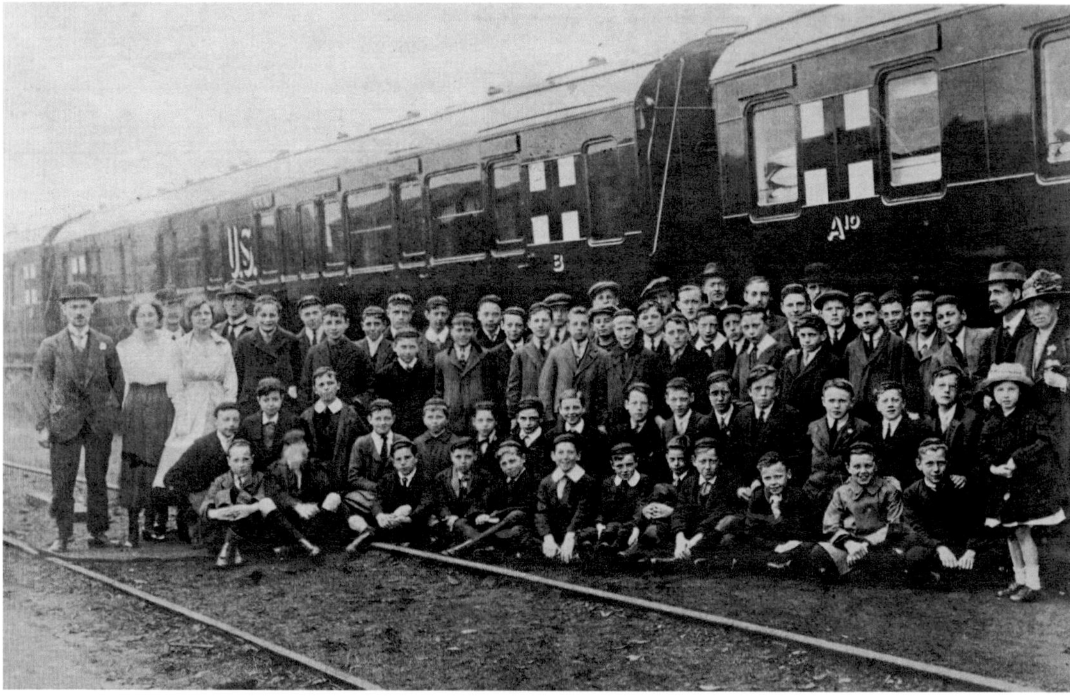

A postcard of a school visit to a US ambulance train at Manchester.

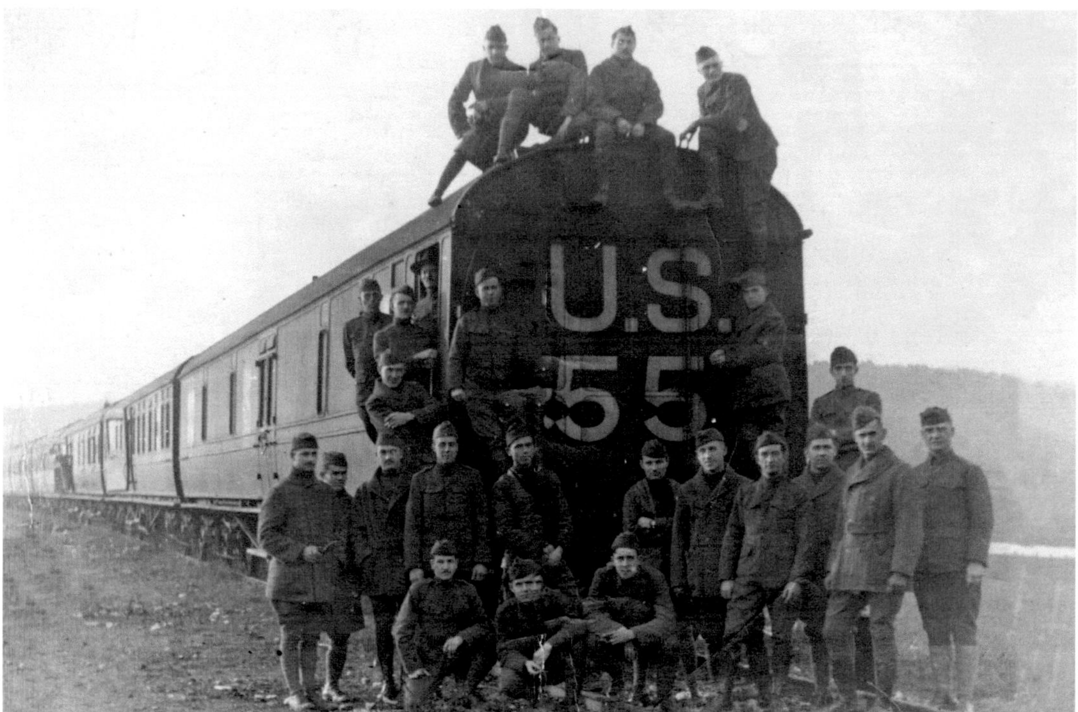

Staff of No. 55 (US) Ambulance Train somewhere in France.

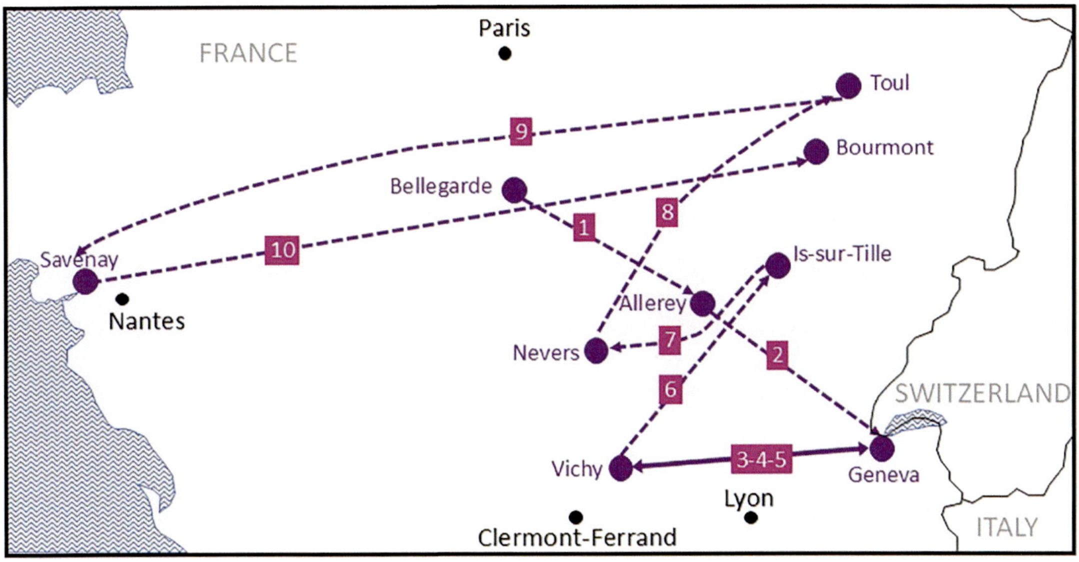

Map showing the journeys of No. 55 (US) Ambulance Train during its last month of operation, December 1918. (Drawn by Sally Finlayson)

Many ambulance trains continued to operate after the Armistice, and it is interesting to look at No. 55 (US) Ambulance Train's final month operating, which was December 1918. The table and map show the ten journeys this train undertook during that month.

No 55 (US) Ambulance Train Movements – Final Month, December 1918					
No.	Date	From	To	Patients	Mileage
1	1st	Bellegarde	Allerey	247	204
2	1st	Allerey	Geneva (Switzerland)		225
3	7th	Geneva (Switzerland)	Vichy	348	259
4	7th	Vichy	Geneva (Switzerland)		259
5	10th	Geneva (Switzerland)	Vichy	316	259
6	12th	Vichy	Is-sur-Tille		210
7	15th	Is-sur-Tille	Nevers		150
8	19th	Nevers	Toul		252
9	21st	Toul	Saveney	442	475
10	22nd	Savenay	Bourmont (Haute Marne)		450

Of particular interest, this train undertook two runs to Geneva in Switzerland. On each occasion the train repatriated over 300 American prisoners of war. During the First World War Switzerland accepted some 68,000 wounded British, French, German and American PoWs. Switzerland remained neutral throughout the war and this was largely respected by the combatants. The servicemen that Switzerland accepted had to have a disability that would negate any further military service.

The historical report ends with a summary of the activity of No. 55 (US) Ambulance Train during the period 1 January 1918 and 1 January 1919 that is tabulated below:

No. 55 (US) Ambulance Train Statistics		
Total number of trips		32
Total number of patients		14,885
Nationalities of patients	American	14,256
	French	345
	British	53
	Belgian	2
	German	229
Average number of patients per trip		465
Total number of miles travelled		16,672
Total number of deaths en route		8
	American	6
	German	2

AMBULANCE TRAINS IN OTHER THEATRES OF THE FIRST WORLD WAR

TOGOLAND

There are records, albeit scant, relating to ambulance trains being operated in various other theatres of the First World War. An expeditionary force of Imperial troops operated against German forces in Togoland, West Africa, between 7 and 26 August 1914. In this short campaign wounded were evacuated from the Battle of Chra by a locally converted ambulance train.[56] This train was fitted out for both lying and sitting casualties at the force base at Lomé but few details have survived.

CAMEROONS

Another expeditionary force consisting of British and French troops moved against German forces in the Cameroons, West Africa, with operations commencing on 26 September 1914.[57] The Cameroons had two railways, and at the beginning of 1915 the Northern Railway was controlled by the British and the French controlled the Midland Railway. Records show that two ambulance rail coaches operated on the Northern Railway and ferried casualties between Edea and Duala, a journey that took four hours.[58]

Six coaches were fitted to take sixteen lying patients and although records state they were used in support of the Western Campaign, it is not clear where they actually operated. What is stated is that these coaches 'proved comfortable and very useful'.[59]

SALONIKA

The Salonika Campaign, also known as the Macedonia Front/Campaign, is often referred to as 'the Forgotten Front' of the First World War. Between 1915 and 1918 British troops were part of an Allied Expeditionary Force fighting the Bulgarian, Austro-Hungarian and German forces in the Balkans. The extremes of climate along with high disease rates amongst the forces posed major problems. The Allies were ultimately successful, and Bulgaria surrendered in September 1918 thus leading to the liberation of Serbia.

In December 1915 the staff for Nos 41 and 42 Ambulance Trains were deployed from England equipped with BDA stretcher frames to install in locally sourced rail wagons.[60] Two Greek ambulance trains consisting of ten wagons each fitted with the Linxweiller stretcher frame system were based in Salonika with one placed at the disposal of British troops.

In June 1916 an ambulance train was assembled based around the above assets, although there appears to be no record as to what number it was allocated or operated under. It consisted of twenty-four assorted vehicles as follows:

1	Kitchen
1	Stores
2	Passenger coaches for staff
10	Greek wagons with the Linxweiller system replaced with BDA
10	Passenger coaches for sitting casualties

The significance of the change to the BDA stretcher frame system was that it increased the capacity of each ambulance wagon from eight to twelve patients.[61] The use of rail for casualty evacuation was effective across the whole area of the campaign but details are fragmented. Much of the fighting took place in isolated locations over difficult terrain and there needed to be much improvisation. In addition, the rail infrastructure was not only standard and broad gauge but there was also a 60 cm narrow-gauge network. Improvised ambulance trains were created from supply trains that had been unloaded in the forward areas. Records show that the broad-gauge improvised trains carried 290 as a mix of sitting and lying patients. Most of the improvised trains were operated by a staff comprising a medical officer and between eight and eleven RAMC other ranks.[62]

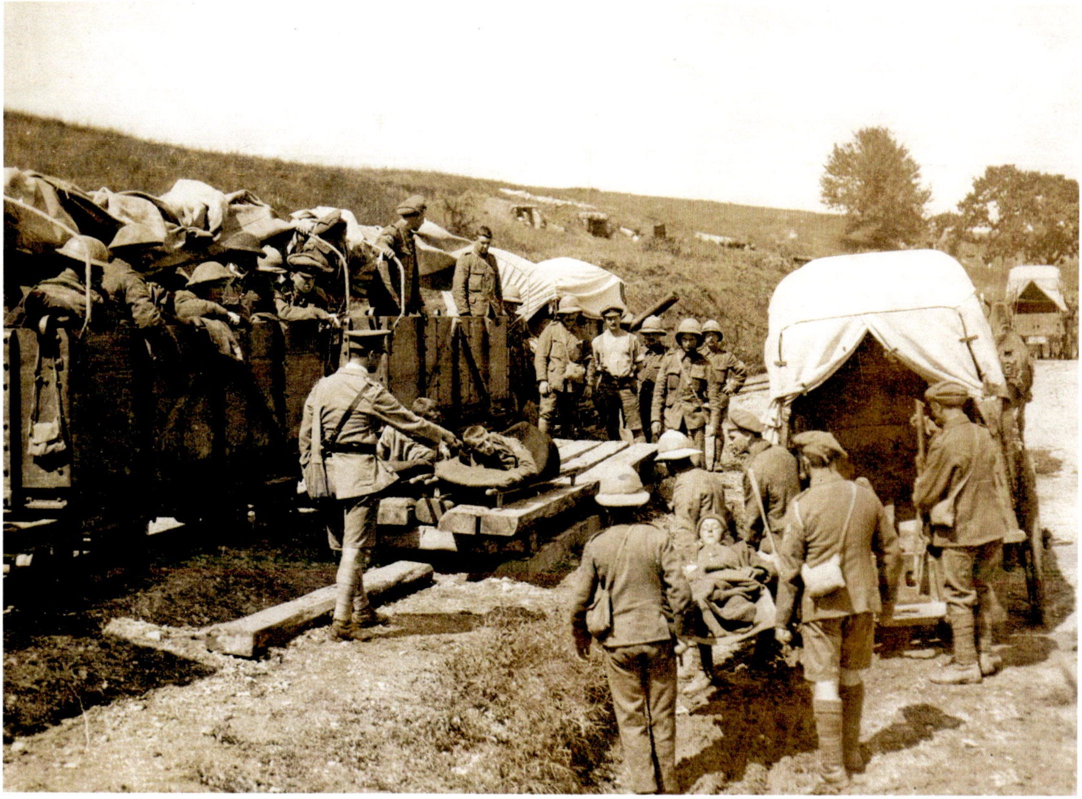

Loading patients on a narrow-gauge railway somewhere on the Salonika Front. (Topical Press Agency)

After the Armistice in 1918 an ambulance train with the capacity of fifty lying and 120 sitting patients was taken over from the Bulgarians and operated by one medical officer and twenty-six RAMC other ranks. This train evacuated patients from Bulgaria to the port of Dedeagatch from which they were transported to Salonika by hospital ship.[63]

Much further east a Russian ambulance train was taken over and operated by the Indian Medical Services and ran from Anenkovo to Krasnovodsk on the eastern side of the Caspian Sea. From there, patients travelled by sea to Baku.[64] Another Russian ambulance train staffed by British Indian personnel operated the Baku–Tiflis–Batoum line.[65]

MESOPOTAMIA

Mesopotamia is a historic region of Asia that covered modern Iraq, although included parts of modern-day Iran, Turkey, Syria and Kuwait. During the First World War British, Australian and Indian troops fought the forces of the Ottoman Empire in a long campaign. There were major medical issues during the campaign, with lack of both resources and clean water leading to high levels of disease.

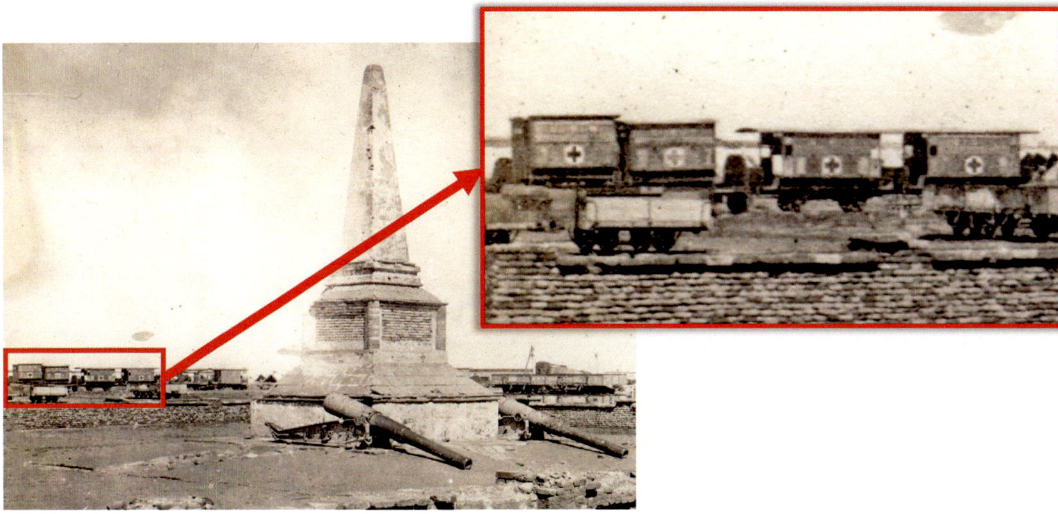

A postcard from Kut in Mesopotamia showing several Baguley-Drewry ambulance railcars.

Two ambulance trains of metre gauge were used in Mesopotamia. Designated A and B, they were initially based at Makina Masus in Basra, with one moved to Baghdad as the war progressed.[66] Train A initially consisted of seven ward coaches, two kitchen cars, a pharmacy car and a baggage wagon. However, it is known that the consist was changed as required.[67]

A fleet of twenty-five 2-ft 6-in-gauge Baguley-Drewry ambulance railcars were ordered by the War Office during 1916 for use on narrow-gauge railways in Mesopotamia, although it is not exactly clear where they operated. The four-wheeled chassis powered with a 20-hp engine were constructed in Burton upon Trent in England and shipped to the Bengal Nagpur Railway in India. Their workshops fitted a unique design of ambulance body that carried six sitting and four stretcher patients.[68, 69]

ITALY

In early 1917 plans were drawn up for an overland supply route from northern France to southern Italy because of the increase in submarine warfare. Known as the Mediterranean Line of Communication (MEDLOC), this approximately 1,400-mile rail route ran from Taranto in southern Italy up the east coast of Italy, then west through Parma and Torino before crossing into France and running north to Cherbourg. Rail expertise was despatched from England and a considerable amount of work was undertaken, including the construction of a marshalling yard at Cherbourg and also a wharf, transit sheds and sidings at Taranto. Camps were also constructed at Cherbourg and St Germain in France along with Faenza and Taranto in Italy where rest, refreshment and sanitary facilities were provided.[70] This MEDLOC route was to carry troop trains, stores and ammunition trains in addition to ambulance trains.

Nos 39 and 43 (Overseas) Ambulance Trains operated this route, and from the summer of 1917 a weekly service would carry some 500 sick and wounded on their journey home. As the war was coming to an end individual ambulance coaches were also added to returning troop trains travelling this MEDLOC route.[71]

Around the time of the Armistice, when four ambulance trains were operating in support of the BEF, there was an increased need for ambulance train capacity. Four additional temporary ambulance trains for sitting patients were created from Italian State Railways rolling stock and operated across northern Italy with RAMC staff. Further trains were needed for a new evacuation route established from Genoa and Marseille in France. This alternative route rejoined the original MEDLOC route at St Germain. In addition, No. 10 Italian Red Cross Train (*X Treno Ospedale*) was made available to the Allies for use on this route.[72] The Sovereign Military Order of Malta provided four hospital trains, as they were described, for use in support of the Italian Army during the course of the war. They were eleven coaches in length and converted from Italian State Railway rolling stock. One SMOM train operated the evacuation route to Marseille.[73]

EGYPT, SINAI AND PALESTINE

The Sinai and Palestine Campaign was part of the Middle Eastern theatre of the First World War and lasted from January 1915 to October 1918. An Egyptian Expeditionary Force along with other Allied forces faced the Central Powers, consisting of the Ottoman Empire, Germany and Austria-Hungary, who had invaded the Sinai Peninsula. The campaign saw the Central Powers pushed back into Palestine and the result was a British and Allied victory. Records show that there were 61,877 British battle casualties along with approximately 6,000 dying of disease and over 100,000 evacuated with diseases. Deaths from disease amongst the Axis forces are recorded at over 40,000.[74] Dysentery, malaria, bilharzia, septic sores, diphtheria, sand-fly fever, scabies and cholera were all to present challenges to the medical services.[75] As with other campaigns, this work will not attempt any detailed description or analysis of the campaign itself but aims to recognise the contribution of ambulance trains.

Following the arrival of the Indian Expeditionary Force in Egypt in December 1915, a total of five ambulance trains were converted in the railway workshops in Cairo from Egyptian State Railways rolling stock. All these trains were to operate west of the Suez Canal. The first three trains were initially designated X, Y and Z according to the Indian Medical Services Units that staffed them but were soon renumbered 1, 2 and 3. The IMS staff were eventually replaced by RAMC personnel in August 1916.

For the planned advance into Palestine, a new railway line was laid by the Royal Engineers across northern Sinai in order to follow the Allied progress into Palestine. The construction of this standard-gauge track was a major engineering task that started at Kantara on the east bank of the Suez Canal and ran east to El Arish and then reached Rafa by the middle of March 1917. A hospital siding was constructed at El Arish so that rail evacuation could be operated in two parts. No ambulance trains crossed the Suez Canal or started operating in the Sinai until December 1917. The Nos 6 and 7 Ambulance Trains commenced operating on this line, with No. 6 working from as near to the front line as possible back to a hospital at El Arish and No. 7 Ambulance Train evacuating west from El Arish to Kantara or Mehamdiya. Macpherson records that there were issues with this line in that it was regularly blocked by sand drifts.[76] From Kantara, two hospital barges were used to cross the Suez Canal, then Nos 1 to 5 Ambulance Trains evacuated patients further west from Kantara West to Alexandria or Port Said to waiting hospital ships.

Medical evacuation following the first Battle of Gaza is documented in detail by Macpherson. The railhead had by this stage reached Khan Yunus and No. 6 Ambulance Train operated from Khan Yunis to Rafa or El Arish, whilst No. 7 operated westwards to Kantara. In addition, improvised trains consisting of covered goods wagons fitted with the BDA apparatus were operated on both sectors of the line. Use was also made of supply wagons returning from the front for the lesser wounded.[77]

The standard-gauge railway that continued to be laid following the Allied advance reached Ludd in January 1918 from where the Allies operated a narrow-gauge line to Jerusalem.[78] As 1918 progressed, the use of rail in Palestine led to an increased need for ambulance trains to operate east of the Suez Canal. The No. 40 Ambulance Train, built by the Midland Railway, was a fifteen-coach train shipped out from England in March 1918 and operated the Kantara to Gaza section of the line. It was considered at the time that three ambulance train journeys per week would prevent the forward hospitals becoming overcrowded.

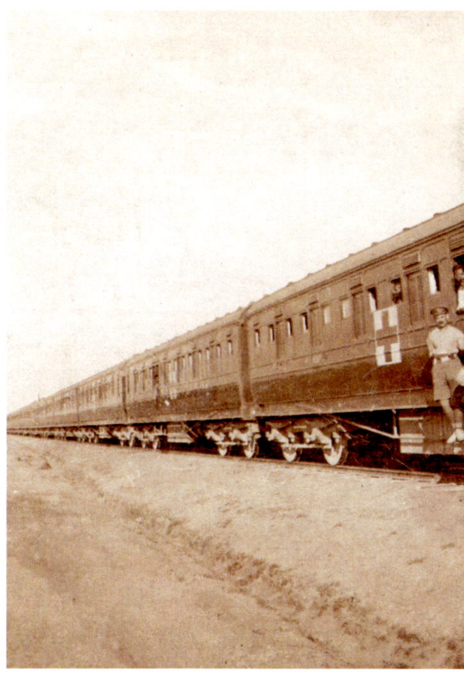

No. 40 Ambulance Train somewhere in the Sinai Peninsula.

It is fair to say that some confusion surrounds the ambulance trains used in Egypt, Sinai and Palestine. For whatever reason, there were several renumberings of the trains and some amalgamation of rolling stock which has led to confusion between the works of different authors. The table below represents a summary that has been assembled from a number of sources.

IMS Unit	Train Number	Entered Service	Eventual Number in 1918	Area of Operation Notes
X	1	December 1914	44	West of Suez
Y	2	December 1914	45	West of Suez
Z	3	December 1914	46	West of Suez
	4 and 5	January 1915	47	West of Suez
	6	December 1916	48	East of Suez
	7	December 1916	49	East of Suez
	8	April 1917	50	East of Suez
	9	June 1917	51	East of Suez
	10	October 1917	56	East of Suez Egyptian casualties and PoWs
	11	?	57	East of Suez Egyptian casualties and PoWs
	40	April 1918	40	Shipped from England

Readers are referred to a very comprehensive article about casualty evacuation in Palestine published in 2020 that reflects much more detailed research into the ambulance trains operating in this campaign.[79]

EAST AFRICA

The East African Campaign of the First World War started in German East Africa and spread to parts of British East Africa, Uganda, Rhodesia, the Belgian Congo and Mozambique. It consisted of a series of battles and guerrilla actions that ran for the whole of the war from 3 August 1914 until 25 November 1918. British forces in East Africa at the start of the war totalled about 1,200. The arrival of the IEF in November 1914 brought an additional 7,000 troops.[80]

Very early in the campaign an ambulance train was organised for the metre-gauge Uganda Railway line from Mombasa to Nairobi. By late 1916 another train was operating on the Maithau to Voi line, the latter being a junction on the Nairobi to Mombasa route. In 1917 with the movement of hostilities further south another

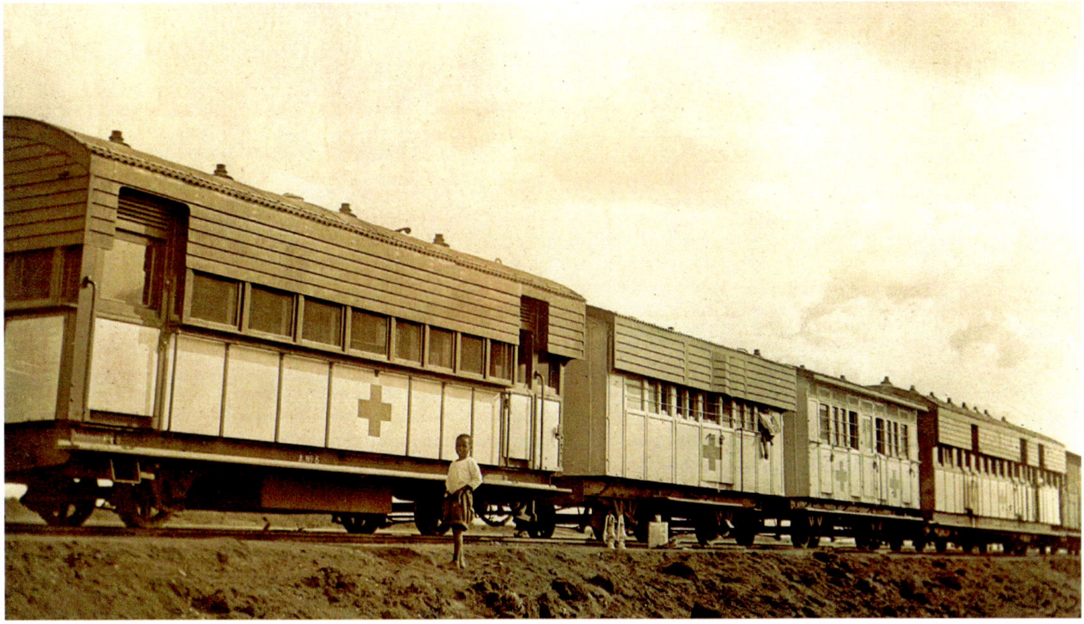

An ambulance train on the Central Railway in East Africa during the First World War.

ambulance train ran on the east–west Central Railway evacuating casualties to hospitals in Dar es Salaam.[81]

NORTH RUSSIA

Starting in March 1918 as the First World War was entering its last few months, the North Russia Intervention was the title history has given to a largely forgotten Allied intervention into the Russian Civil War. A force comprising British, American, French, Italian, Polish and Czechoslovakian troops was sent to north Russia in support of the White Russian resistance against the Bolsheviks following the Russian Revolution. This force operated south from the Murmansk and Archangel regions of north Russia.

Early in the deployment an improvised ambulance train of 100 beds and a combined disinfection and bath train is recorded as being stationed at Obozerskaya, approximately 100 miles south of Archangel, although sadly no operational details have survived.[82] Disinfection and bath trains either separately or in combination were to be found in other countries during the First World War, most notably in Austro-Hungary.

By August 1919 two British ambulance trains were in operation on the Murman Railway. Designated 60 and 61 Ambulance Trains, they should not be confused with the No. 60 (US) and No. 61 (US) Ambulance Trains operated by American troops on the Western Front in Europe. Very little detail seems to have survived about these two north Russian trains except that No. 61 operated as far as possible towards the front line with the Bolshevik forces and evacuated patients back to Kem. The front line was some 500 miles in length and encircled Archangel on three sides. No. 60 ambulance train operated from Kem north to the port of Murmansk.[83]

The North Russian Intervention Force was deployed for some nineteen months until a decision was made by the various Allied governments to withdraw from Russia in October 1919.

AMBULANCE TRAIN COMFORT FUNDS

As has been described earlier, funds were raised from the public by the exhibiting of ambulance trains around the country prior to being shipped to France. More than 18,000 charities were established to help the war effort in various ways during the First World War.[84] The most popular causes were to provide 'comforts' for the troops such as clothing, books, food and cigarettes. Local authorities around the country organised comfort funds for soldiers and sailors, and there were also knitting groups providing items such as gloves and socks. These funds not only sent items to troops abroad but some also provided help for families back home.

Other countries who provided troops to the war also had comfort funds to support their servicemen. The Australian Comfort Fund is stated to have provided 12 million mugs of tea to soldiers during the course of the First World War.[85]

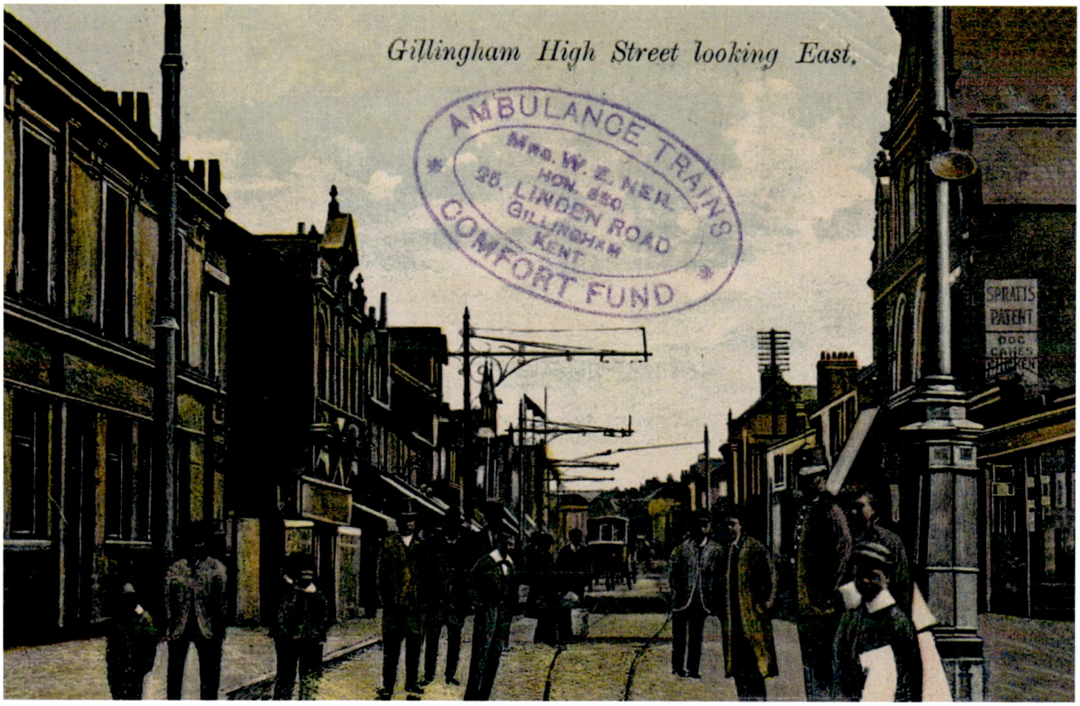

A postcard of Gillingham, Kent, carrying the handstamp of an 'AMBULANCE TRAIN COMFORT FUND' and posted from Brighton.

The picture postcard of Gillingham in Kent opposite was posted on 25 November 1917 and carries the handstamp of an Ambulance Train Comfort Fund that was also based in Gillingham. The implication of this card is that it was provided to returning troops to write and then post on their arrival at their destination hospital. This card was subsequently posted from Brighton and the writer informs his family that he is in 'Kitchener's Hospital, Block B2, Ward 9, Brighton'.

Gillingham and other Kent towns initially had a role receiving casualties by ambulance trains that had started operating out of Southampton from October 1914. These trains would have been operated by the LSWR and handed over to the SECR at Guildford. After hospital ships started arriving at Dover Marine from January 1915 the procedure would have reversed, although it is not clear whether the soldier who wrote the card had arrived at Dover or Chatham. The ambulance train likely to have been carrying him would have been handed over to the LBSCR at Guildford to be worked forward to Brighton.

The author of the card made reference to going to the Kitchener hospital in Brighton. This hospital opened in 1915 and was the largest of three hospitals for Indian troops in Brighton with over 1,700 beds. When the majority of the Indian Army was sent to Mesopotamia and Egypt, the Canadians took over the Kitchener military hospital on 14 March 1917. It was formally designated the 10th Canadian General Hospital from 10 September 1917 and was eventually handed back to the RAMC on 13 March 1919.

It is therefore likely that the author of this card who was supported by this Ambulance Train Comfort Fund was admitted to the 10th Canadian General Hospital in Brighton on or just before 25 November 1917.

There were other welfare services for troops travelling on ambulance trains, as evidenced by a postcard that was posted from Banbury in Oxfordshire on 21 September 1918. The card carries the heading of 'BANBURY G.W.R. REST STATION' with a central Red Cross along with a strapline of 'Refreshments for Sick and Wounded Soldiers and Sailors'. The writer states: 'I arrived at Southampton this morning. Cannot say where I am being sent to now by train to hospital.'

4
Second World War

Many authors have commented on how much less information is readily available, or has indeed survived, concerning ambulance train operations during the Second World War as compared with the First World War.[1] References have been seen in relation to individual operations that simply state that casualties were moved by rail, with no details as to the organisation and staffing of the trains utilised. Mention was made earlier of ambulance train postal history, and it is also the case that far less has survived from the Second World War than the First. One reason is that during the First World War many hundreds of thousands of postcards were sent but by the Second World War these were being replaced by letters where the envelopes tended not to survive.

The operating of ambulance trains in the Second World War will be considered under several headings in a similar way to the First World War. There was a major difference with the provision of casualty evacuation trains (CETs) in addition to both home and overseas ambulance trains. Trains were, once again, produced for use by the US Army after they entered the war, and another difference was that they operated ambulance trains both in England before D-Day and overseas after D-Day.

It is well known that the National Health Service in the United Kingdom came into being after the Second World War on 5 July 1948. However, with the likelihood of war in Europe the government created the Emergency Hospital Service in 1939. This was later renamed the Emergency Medical Services and its aim was to give central government control over all types of hospitals both voluntary and municipal so as to manage the anticipated influx of casualties. The Emergency Medical Services did not only encompass hospitals, but included Civil Defence services, ambulances and ambulance trains along with river ambulances on the River Thames that were part of the Port of London Authority's River Emergency Service. A very detailed two-volume history of all aspects of the Emergency Medical Services in the Second World War was published in 1951.[2]

Mention should be made of a very important primary source of information related to British ambulance trains that has been made available to the author. The late Lt Col (retd) Leonard Hudson MBE had a career in British Rail for forty-seven years and during the Second World War was seconded to the Movements Directorate of the War Office, his department being Q(M)4. In his own words he was '...asked to co-ordinate all rail movements of personnel and unit vehicles and baggage within the UK'. The military ambulance trains fell within this remit and from March 1944 the control of the CETs was transferred from the Ministry of Health to Q(M)4. Two other trains fell within Lt Col Hudson's extensive remit, and these were the Supreme Commander Allied Expeditionary Force, General Dwight D. Eisenhower's train codenamed ALIVE, along with the British Prime Minister Winston Churchill's train codenamed RUGGED.

In 1992 Lt Col Hudson provided the author with a copy of papers he had drafted and submitted in 1946 for the historical record of movements during the war. These personal papers will be drawn on heavily for the home ambulance train story, and in particular the preparations for D-Day.[3]

Following Germany's invasion of Poland, Great Britain and France declared war on Germany on 3 September 1939. By October 1939, thirty-four casualty evacuation trains had been prepared by various railway companies, and by spring 1940 twenty-five ambulance trains had been converted of which twelve were ready for use at home and thirteen for use overseas.[4] Many more trains were converted as the need increased as well as those required for use by American Forces once they arrived in Europe. There has been considerable confusion over the detail and numbering of Second World War ambulance trains but it is hoped that this work goes some way to offering a definitive statement as to the British ambulance train assets that were available.

CASUALTY EVACUATION TRAINS

The work of preparing rolling stock for casualty evacuation was commenced by the Home Office in April 1939 in collaboration with the Ministry of Transport and the War Office.[5] Once commissioned the casualty evacuation trains were initially placed under the management of the Ministry of Health and under the operational direction of the Director General of the Emergency Medical Services.

The Great Western Railway produced the initial six CETs that comprised twelve vehicles each, nine of which were Siphon G milk vans. These early conversions were very spartan and carried forty-three stretchers per van. The other three vehicles in each train were two brake vans and a corridor coach for staff. All thirty-four CETs were produced to the same specifications and were ready for deployment on 4 September 1939. In all some 564 vehicles were converted to form the CETs by a number of different railway workshops.

When first introduced it was envisaged that the CETs would be utilised in the event of the widespread bombing of British cities. They were never actually used in that role, although they contributed to the evacuation of London hospitals, as will be described below. In fact, by December 1939 their number was reduced to eighteen. Some of the released vehicles were subsequently incorporated into overseas ambulance trains.

As in the First World War, confusion over train numbers occurred and one thing done to alleviate this was that the thirty-four CETs were renumbered prefixing with 3 to become 301–34 (inclusive). There were five stabling railheads allocated to CETs and each had a nominated alternative in case of infrastructure problems. In the early stages of the war the CETs were allocated to Tunbridge Wells, Sevenoaks, Tattenham Corner, Hassocks and Earley.[6]

The staff of a CET was led by a medical officer supplied by the Central Medical Service Committee. Initially there was also a Hospital Transport Officer, which was an administrative role, but subsequently withdrawn. There were two nursing sisters provided by the Civil Nursing Reserve along with ten auxiliary nurses and eight orderlies, the latter being supplied by the SJAB.[7] Sources often refer to the CETs as ambulance trains but they were quite separate from the home ambulance trains. One major distinguishing feature was that the HATs displayed the Red Cross emblem on the roof and sides of the coaches whereas the CETs did not.

The CETs played a major role in the evacuation of London hospitals in preparation of the anticipated large-scale bombing. Instructions were issued in July 1944 and the evacuations took place during August with sixty-eight CET journeys carrying

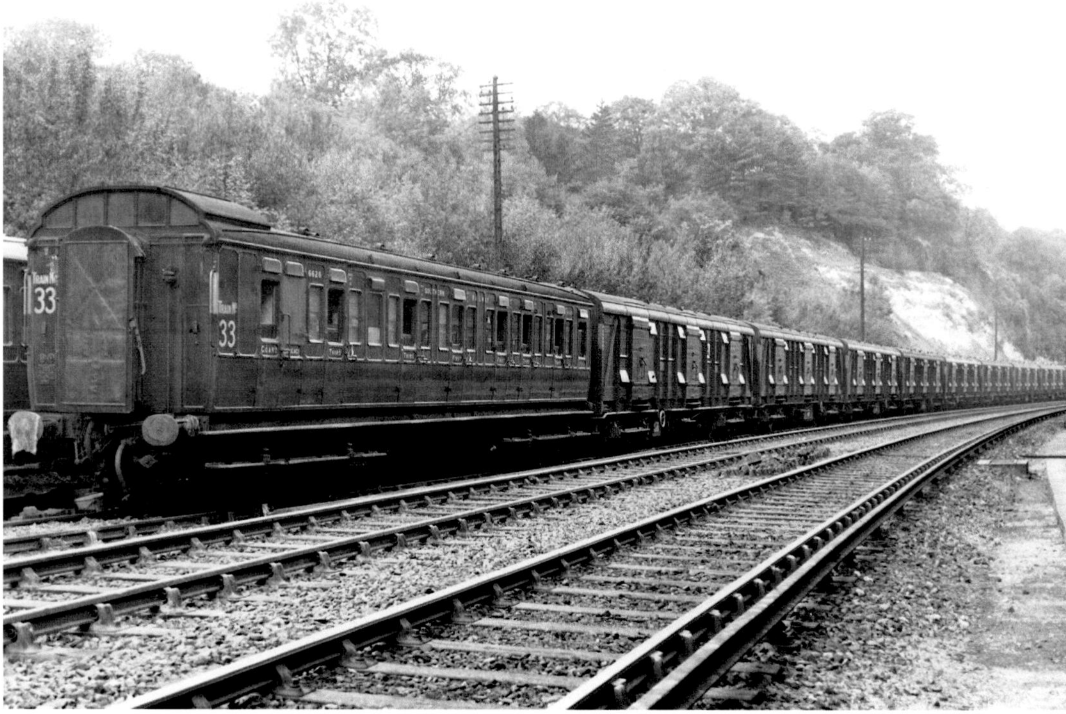

No. 33 Casualty Evacuation Train, October 1939. (Alamy)

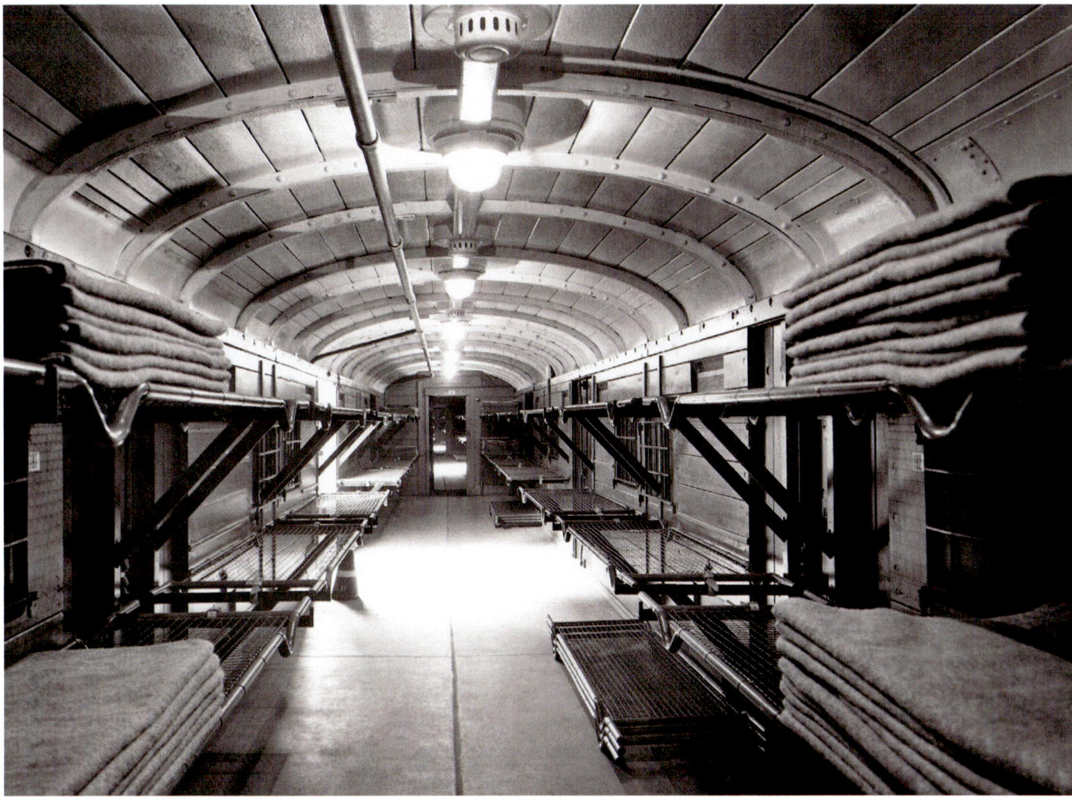

The interior of No. 33 CET, October 1939. (Alamy)

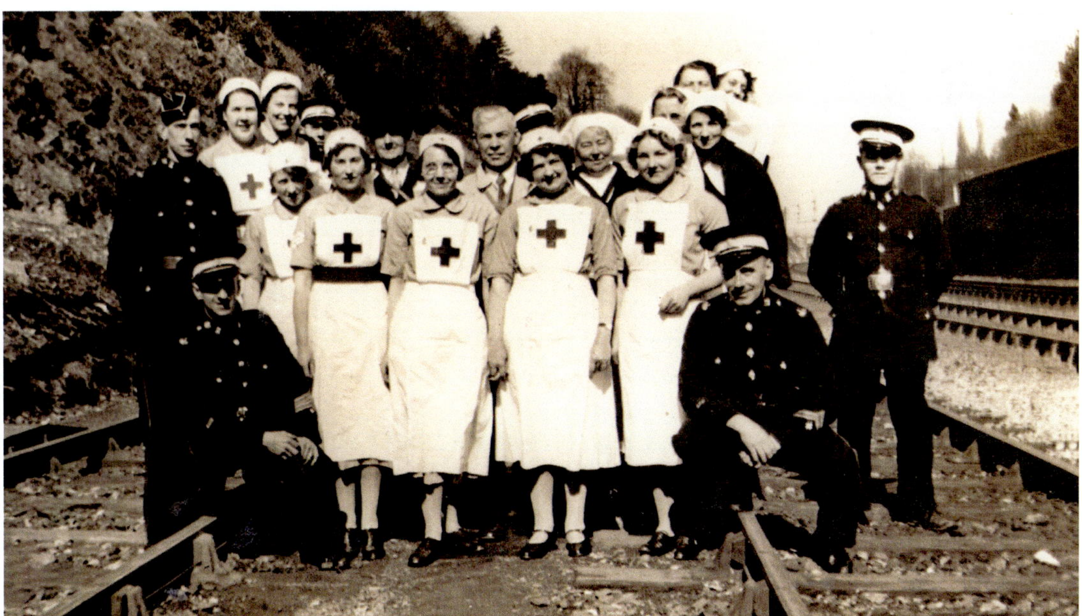

Staff of No. 34 CET at Sevenoaks.

13,152 patients.[8] Patients were entrained at two stations, Addison Road, now modern-day Kensington Olympia, and Marylebone. Stretcher bearers were provided by the newly formed Army Pioneer Corps that had been raised in 1939 and was to be given a 'Royal' title in 1946 in recognition of their contribution to the war effort. The RPC was subsequently amalgamated into the Royal Logistic Corps in 1993.

HOME AMBULANCE TRAINS

By the outbreak of the war the War Office was provided with eight ambulance trains that were converted by the LMS Railway. They were each nine vehicles in length and had a capacity of 120 lying and 40 sitting casualties. These HATs were initially numbered 1 to 8 but were later changed to 55 to 62 (inclusive) as the overseas ambulance trains were also numbered 1 to 8. They were initially stabled at Newhaven and Seaford in East Sussex as it was anticipated that casualties from the BEF would arrive via Newhaven.

On 8 November 1939 a Committee that would oversee all aspects of supply and maintenance of ambulance trains sat for the first time. This Committee comprised a range of organisations so that all issues could be dealt with in one forum. Although not all were members from the beginning, the Committee eventually consisted of representatives from the Ministries of Transport, Supply and Health, the Railway Executive Committee, the War Office, Admiralty and Air Ministry, the Southern Railway, Great Western Railway, London, Midland & Scottish Railway and London & North Eastern Railway along with the US Army. At that first meeting a decision was made to increase the sitting casualty capacity to 152 per train by adding two open third-class coaches. Also, four additional HATs to be numbered 63 to 66 (inclusive) were requested. The table below details the delivery dates and the initial allocation of these twelve HATs.

Train Number	Delivery Date	Initial Stabling Point	Stabling Point from 16 January 1940
55	20 September 1939	Newhaven	Southampton
56	20 September 1939	Newhaven	Southampton
57	7 October 1939	Newhaven	Southampton
58	20 October 1939	Newhaven	Southampton
59	24 October 1939	Newhaven	Newhaven
60	28 October 1939	Newhaven	Newhaven
61	1 November 1939	Newhaven	Newhaven
62	25 October 1939	Newhaven	Newhaven
63	13 April 1940	Southampton	Southampton
64	13 April 1940	Southampton	Southampton
65	18 May 1940	Bournemouth	Bournemouth
66	18 May 1940	Bournemouth	Bournemouth

Inevitably the stabling points of trains changed depending on need, and in particular trains were re-allocated during 1940 following the evacuation from Dunkirk. Five trains were reserved for the reception of casualties at ports following long sea journeys from various theatres of the war with seven trains being held for movements around the country. The table below shows the trains reserved for port use along with their stabling points.

Train Number	New Stabling Point	Date of Move	Port Served
56	Ruabon, North Wales	29 June 1940	Liverpool
57	Bellahouston, Glasgow	15 August 1940	Glasgow
58	Steeps Road, Glasgow	15 August 1940	Glasgow
60	Blackpool	4 July 1940	Liverpool
65	Weston-super-Mare	18 August 1940	Avonmouth

These five trains were to remain based at these stabling points until just before D-Day when several more re-allocations were undertaken. The mention of Ruabon in the above table as a stabling point may seem a bit strange as today this station is an unstaffed halt on the Shrewsbury to Chester line. However, the station was originally much larger and had an extensive marshalling yard and goods depot with an associated turntable, so it was clearly fit for purpose as an ambulance train stabling point.

An RAMC veteran who served on No. 65 HAT provided the author with some personal recollections.[9] He first joined the train when it was stabled at Bournemouth West and collected wounded from Southampton Docks following the Dunkirk evacuation. In common with many of the ambulance trains after the evacuation of Dunkirk there were a number of reallocations of stabling points around the country. No. 65 HAT was moved to the Locking Road Station at Weston-super-Mare on 18 August 1940 from where it was to service Avonmouth Docks in Bristol. The reminiscences describe wounded collected from Avonmouth as coming from the North African Campaign. There were long periods of inactivity awaiting the arrival of hospital ships and the train staff relieved the boredom by helping local farmers with their potato harvesting and were even allowed to attend tea-dances at the Winter Gardens in Weston-super-Mare.

July 1942 saw two nights of heavy bombing of Weston-super-Mare in which the railway goods yard was targeted but the train and its staff escaped unscathed. Ambulance train staff had previously been given instruction in uncoupling coaches and on these nights they were able to isolate some burning GWR coaches thus avoiding the spread of fire. No. 65 HAT was to remain stabled at and operating out of Weston-super-Mare until Operation OVERLORD and D-Day.

The remaining seven HATs were utilised as required for internal patient movement throughout the country. The Hudson Papers give a rare insight into the movements of these trains prior to D-Day, as shown in the table below.

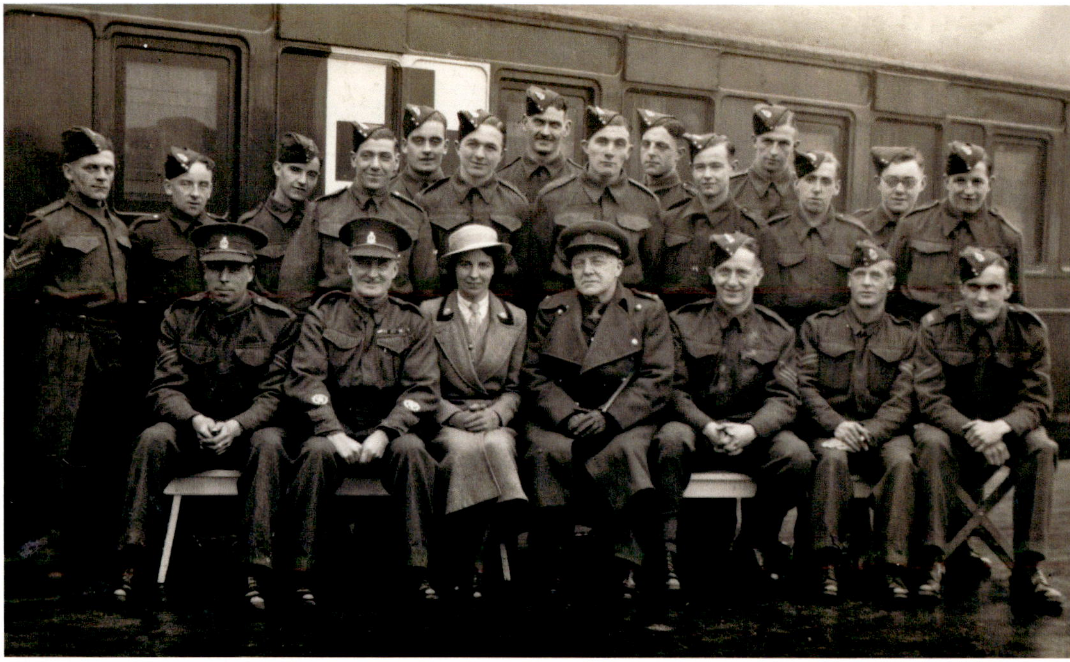

Staff of No. 65 (Home) Ambulance Train at Weston-super-Mare in January 1941. (F. T. Holt)

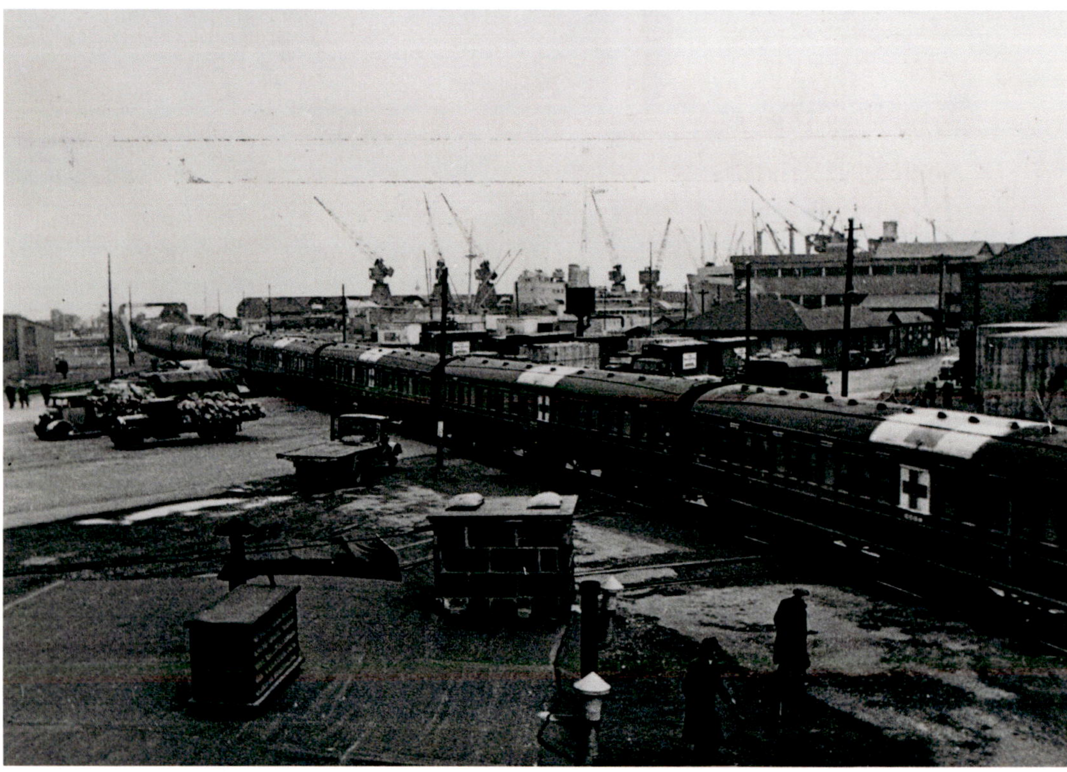

A home ambulance train at Avonmouth Docks in March 1944. (Bristol Archives ref: 42242/Ph/3/18)

Train Number	Stabling Points	Date of Moves
55	Hanwood	20 September 1940
59	Burton upon Trent	1 July 1940
61	Kidlington	3 July 1940
62	Three Bridges	5 June 1940
	Bracknell	8 July 1940
	Horley	2 April 1941
	Tattenham Corner	22 April 1941
63	Market Harborough	3 July 1940
	Hassocks	17 November 1941
64	Bournemouth	11 June 1940
	Market Harborough	3 July 1940
	Loughborough	11 May 1942
	Lincoln (LMS)	27 October 1943
66	Aberdare	18 August 1940

This table has much to interest local historians with its now disused stations, lifted railway infrastructure and redeveloped good yards. For example, the Lincoln (LMS station) referred to was Lincoln St Marks which closed in 1985. Another avenue of research is the correlation between these various stations and the hospitals large and small, municipal or military that they served. How many communities today will be aware of the important role their local railway station may have played during either world war?

Ten additional ambulance trains had been requested in early 1940, although only eight were actually delivered. Hudson records that they were never brought into full use. However, Nos 67 and 68 were subsequently allocated to the two HATs in Northern Ireland.

Train Number	Stabling Points
67	Langley
68	Langley
69	Renumbered to MoH CET No. 311
70	Renumbered to MoH CET No. 313
71	Langley
72	Willesden
73	Willesden
74	Swindon
75	Swindon
76	Sevenoaks

The USA entered the war on 8 December 1941. The first American troops arrived in Great Britain in January 1942 and set about the organisation and training that was to lead up to the eventual invasion of Europe on D-Day as part of Operation OVERLORD. As in the First World War, railway companies converted rolling stock for use by the US Army both within Great Britain and eventually in Continental Europe.

The first ambulance train for American use was converted by GWR and handed over at a press launch on 25 March 1943. This train consisted of fourteen carriages with a patient lift of between 250 to 317 depending on the mix of stretcher and walking patients. This initial train was mainly used for training and the first operational train was handed over on 2 June 1943. By September 1943 the US Army had fifteen ambulance trains operating within Great Britain.

In July 1943 the US Army requested five additional ambulance trains to staff and use to support the US hospitals being established around the country. The most expeditious way to accede to this request was to hand over five of the HATs that were already fully equipped and operational. The five trains and their handover dates are detailed in the table below.

Train Number	Stabling Points	Date of Handover
55	Blinkhorn, Taunton	27 December 1943
57	Malvern Wells	27 December 1943
59	Swindon Junction	15 November 1943
61	Sudbury, Staffordshire	9 August 1943
64	Newbury	15 November 1943

The GWR also provided the Americans with four coaches and two storage vans for use as an ambulance train maintenance unit, although it is not known where they were stabled.

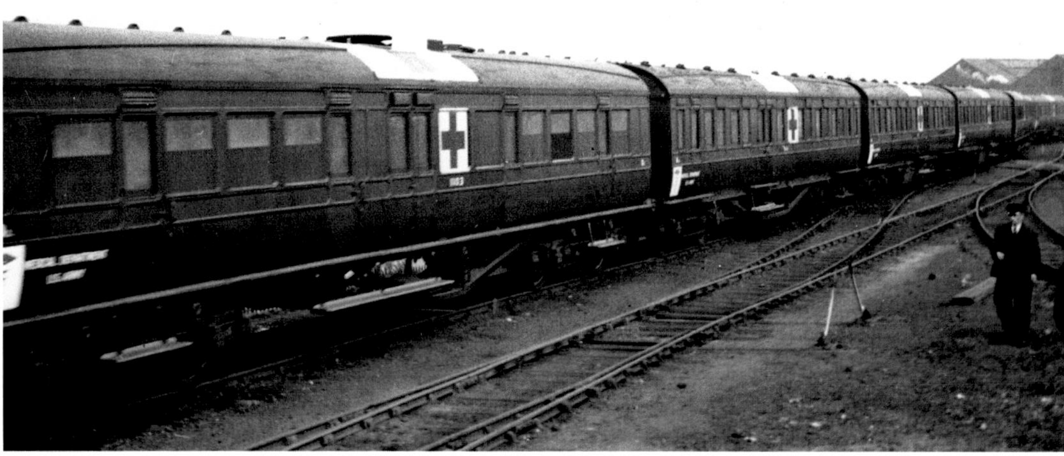

The handover on 25 March 1943 of the first ambulance train converted by GWR for use by the US Army. (Topical Press Agency)

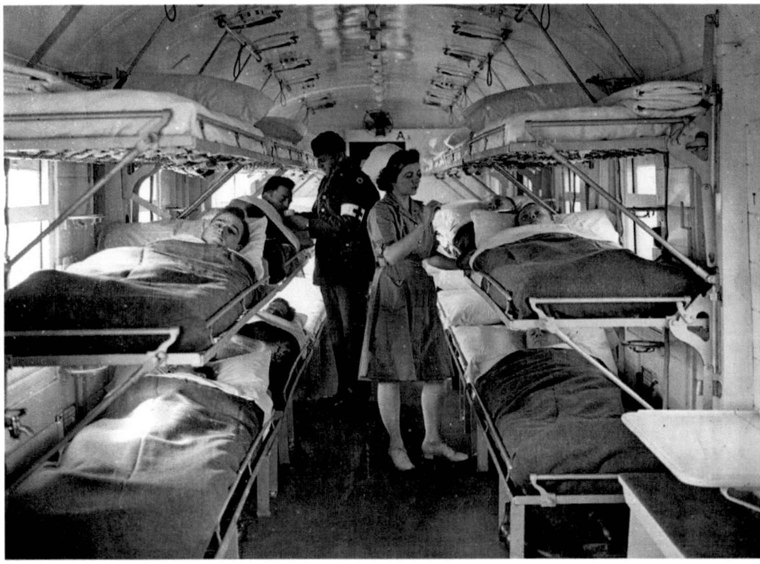

One of the ward coaches at the press launch and handover of the first ambulance train to the US Army. (Topical Press Agency)

In late 1943 the HATs were to contribute to the repatriation of British PoWs. On 25 October 1943 two ships, SS *Drottningholm* and RMS *Empress of Russia*, arrived at Leith in Scotland. SS *Drottningholm* was one of the earliest steam turbine ocean liners and was built and launched in Scotland in 1904 as RMS *Virginian*. It was sold to the Swedish American Line and renamed in 1920. The link with neutral Sweden meant that during the Second World War it was recognised as a neutral passenger ship and used to repatriate civilians and PoWs to a number of different countries. RMS *Empress of Russia* was another ocean liner built in 1912 also in Scotland. It had sailed from Gothenburg in Sweden to Leith. Another ship, HMHS *Atlantis*, also repatriated PoWs to Liverpool the following day. Over those two days the distribution of these returning servicemen required nine of the twelve HATs, as shown in the table below.

Train Number	Total Carried	From	To
55	350	Leith Dock	Netley
57	220	Leith Dock	Turnberry
58	304	Leith Dock	Kingston upon Thames
59	250	Liverpool	Watford
60	250	Leith Dock	Manchester
62	304	Leith Dock	Kingston upon Thames
63	250	Leith Central	Surbiton
64	350	Leith Dock	Bedford
66	200	Liverpool	Netley

One aspect that posed difficulties for HATs was the provision of stretcher bearers to unload trains. Initially these were found by the MoH hospitals but there were issues with availability. The War Office agreed to supply stretcher bearers at the detraining stations from the nearest military training depots with the civilian services providing the necessary transport.[10]

In the latter years of the war twelve LSWR dining saloons were converted into self-contained ambulance cars for use when full-size ambulance trains were not appropriate. They were mainly used by the US Army, although one was utilised by the Royal Navy.[11]

Mention should be made of home ambulance trains in Northern Ireland. By the commencement of the Second World War Ireland had been partitioned for some eighteen years. Two ambulance trains were provided in Northern Ireland, initially numbered 14 and 15. Several of the required coaches were provided by the LMS and re-bogied to the Irish rail gauge. Both trains had thirteen vehicles, and No. 15 included four vans that had been in No. 13 Ambulance Train in Ireland during the First World War.

Initially operated by the RAMC, both trains were taken over by the US No. 44 Hospital Train Unit. In late 1943, as already mentioned and to avoid confusion, the two trains were renumbered 67 and 68 HATs respectively.[12] Both trains were initially based at Whitehead on the east coast of County Antrim but No. 15 was subsequently moved to Broomhedge near Lisburn. Neither train was used for any battle casualties, but they did move patients between military hospitals within Northern Ireland.[13]

OVERSEAS AMBULANCE TRAINS

As in the First World War, the various railway companies all contributed to the production of overseas ambulances trains. There was one major difference in that all the design work was done by the LMS and individual railway companies were responsible for one type of vehicle conversion. These were then sent to a central point to be marshalled into trains. The LMS also procured all the materials that were needed and forwarded them to the workshops concerned.[14]

In Europe, the story of overseas British Army ambulance trains is divided into two distinct periods. Firstly, the British Expeditionary Force, mobilised to France in September 1939 and its subsequent retreat and evacuation from Dunkirk as Operation DYNAMO. Secondly, there was the preparation for Operation OVERLORD and D-Day, in June 1944, following which ambulance train operations in Europe recommenced and continued to evacuate wounded until the end of hostilities and beyond.

THE BRITISH EXPEDITIONARY FORCE AND OPERATION DYNAMO

Mention was made earlier that thirteen ambulance trains were converted for use overseas but initially only nine were shipped to France in support of the BEF.

In the first weeks of operation of the BEF sick and wounded were admitted to French civilian hospitals prior to British general hospitals being deployed across the Channel.[15] Prior to the arrival of the nine trains, the French made four ambulance trains available for the use of the BEF. These were two *trains sanitaires couché*, which carried 300 lying patients each, and two *trains sanitaires mixte*, carrying 120 lying and 240 sitting patients each.[16]

The nine trains of the BEF were numbered 51–54, 5–8 and 10. Trains 9 and 11 were completed too late for shipment. For some reason train 10 was renumbered 13. They were sixteen coaches in length and hauled by a French locomotive. Each train had a staff of three medical officers, three nursing sisters and forty-five other ranks.

In January 1940 an Ambulance Train Maintenance Company RE was formed to support the BEF ambulance trains in France.[17] Presumably part of this maintenance company, No. 1 and No. 2 Ambulance Train Maintenance Sections are recorded as being located at Dieppe and Étaples respectively.[18] Records exist of the various Railway Construction Companies (RCC) that were sent out with the BEF, one of whose roles was the construction of sidings for airfield sites in northern France. In early May 1940, 151 RCC is recorded as building sidings specifically for ambulance trains at Étaples.[19]

It was reported that these early overseas ambulance trains had two major issues, namely water supply and heating. Although water was plentiful, a hose had been omitted from the scale of equipment of each train resulting in considerable effort by the staff using buckets. Heating for a train was provided by steam from the locomotive being driven through pipes throughout the train.[20] On occasions, when the locomotive left the train the rolling stock could become extremely cold with steam pipes freezing. There were also incompatibilities between French locomotives and British rolling stock that could lead to harsh braking and problems climbing gradients.

The withdrawal of the BEF back to the Dunkirk region and its eventual evacuation between 26 May and 6 June 1940, Operation DYNAMO, is well documented in many histories. What is less well known are the valiant efforts made by the available ambulance trains to transport wounded back to the coast in the hope that they could be moved across the Channel. There are accounts of ambulance trains coming under fire on their way to Dieppe and Dunkirk irrespective of the presumed protection of the Red Cross displayed on the carriages. One train loaded with casualties and some 40 miles from Dunkirk apparently took three days to complete the journey.[21] Trains were brought to a standstill by damaged track and abandoned rolling stock. No. 6 (Overseas) Ambulance Train was one such train that became stranded, with blown-up track to both front and rear. Sadly, it was never to reach the coast and all on board became PoWs.[22] Four ambulance trains – Nos 5, 6, 7 and 8 – were lost at Dunkirk but some stock remained in France only to be recommissioned after D-Day several years later.[23]

One of the ambulance trains operating with the BEF was No. 13 and a group photograph of the staff has survived. The photograph carries the inscription 'No 13 Ambulance Train. France. Belgium. Dunkirk. May 1940'. It is annotated on the

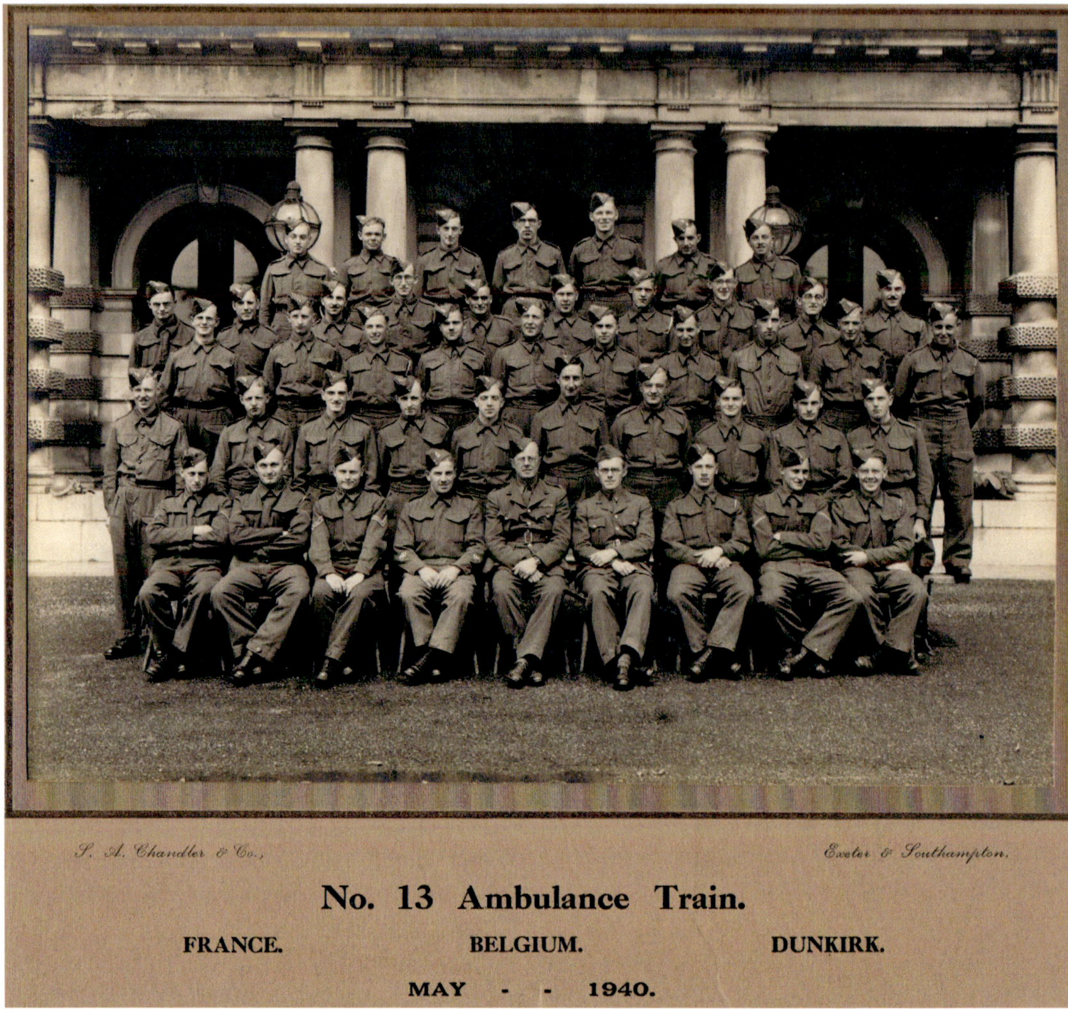

A group photograph of No. 13 (Overseas) Ambulance Train staff taken at the Royal Victoria Hospital, Netley, after return from Dunkirk.

reverse with the names of the staff and also states 'Photograph taken at Netley Hospital, approximately August 1940 prior to disbanding'. This is a reference to the Royal Victoria Hospital, Netley, in Hampshire and it appears that other ambulance train staff returning from the BEF after the Dunkirk evacuation were also sent there. A piece of postal history that has survived is an envelope posted from Richmond, Surrey, some five days before the Dunkirk evacuation and addressed to a member of the staff on No. 7 Ambulance Train. This was returned undeliverable after Dunkirk and redirected to '7th Ambulance Train, Netley'.

To complete the Operation DYNAMO story, 338,226 Allied troops are recorded as having been rescued from the beaches of Dunkirk by a large flotilla of ships of all types and sizes, from naval vessels of many types to the legendary fleet of 'little ships'.[24] Of relevance to this work, forty-seven ambulance train journeys

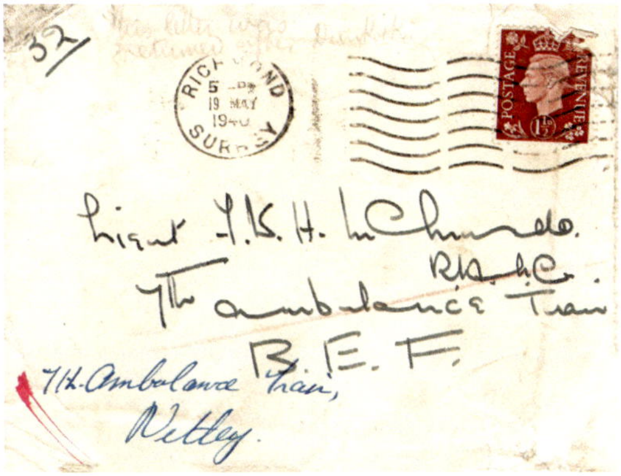

An envelope posted from Surrey in May 1940 to an ambulance train of the BEF and returned as a consequence of the Dunkirk evacuation. It is marked to be redirected to the Royal Victoria Hospital, Netley.

transported 28,354 wounded having been landed at Dover, Margate, Newhaven and Ramsgate, to hospitals inland.[25, 26]

OPERATION OVERLORD AND D-DAY

Operation OVERLORD was the overall Allied plan to reoccupy France and eventually liberate Europe. It was initiated on D-Day, 6 June 1944, which was part of Operation NEPTUNE, more commonly referred to as the Normandy landings or the Allied invasion of Normandy. In late 1943 detailed planning commenced for the reception of casualties from Operation OVERLORD and changes were made in both the hospital service along with reallocations of ambulance trains in preparation for the anticipated influx of casualties.

Agreement was reached on the various ports for the reception of casualties as in the table below.

Port	Vessels	Responsibility
Tilbury	Hospital ships Hospital carriers Landing Ship Tank (LSTs)	British
Portsmouth	Hospital carriers	British
Gosport	LSTs	British
Southampton	Hospital ships Hospital carriers LSTs	Joint
Portland	LSTs	American
Weymouth	LSTs	American
Plymouth	Hospital ships Hospital carriers LSTs	American
Avonmouth	Hospital ships	Joint

Mention should be made of the difference between a hospital ship and a hospital carrier in that more specialised conversion was undertaken to create hospital ships, although both sailed under the Red Cross emblem. During the Second World War over 1,000 of the very versatile Landing Ship Tank (LST) were produced. Once they had delivered vehicles, troops and stores ashore, they became the primary casualty transport back to England. Following D-Day, by September 1944 LSTs had returned 41,035 wounded across the Channel.[27]

It was agreed that no attempt would be made to segregate casualties be they British, Canadian, American or PoWs until they reached one of the transit hospitals established across southern England. One such example of the changes made to a hospital was Park Prewett Hospital in Basingstoke which also serves as a good example of the integration of rail into the plans.[28] The instructions issued to Park Prewett Hospital were that its role was to change from a general to a transit hospital. It would increase in size and receive additional staff. Casualties would arrive by ambulance trains from south coast ports and patients would be detained at the SR siding at Basingstoke Station, with forty-eight RAMC personnel made available as stretcher bearers. Records show that seventy-one ambulance trains were received at Basingstoke from south coast ports.

One of the roles of a transit hospital was to sort casualties into their nationalities so that when fit Canadian patients, for example, could be transferred to Canadian hospitals and likewise American patients moved to American hospitals around the country. After D-Day, to make these patient transfers happen, sixty-one ambulance train journeys were recorded as having been undertaken from Basingstoke to base hospitals in the Midlands and north of England.

In preparation for D-Day a total of forty-four ambulance trains were available for use in Great Britain. These included the MoH CETs whose control was transferred to the War Office Q(M)4. The other ambulance train assets were the HATs operated by both the British and American armies along with eleven American OATs that were operating in Great Britain before being shipped across to France.

Eight of the CETs were dedicated to transfers from ports to transit hospitals, with the other trains distributing casualties to base hospitals around the country. In the weeks and months that followed D-Day, various trains were decommissioned in response to the workload, as shown in the table below. Records show that by the time they were all disbanded in 1945 the CETs had carried 192,557 patients of whom 152,492 were British, American and Canadian troops.[29]

British CETs	Date Withdrawn	Notes
101	16 June 1945	Originally built for the BEF but too late to be shipped
102	21 June 1945	
301	14 July 1945	
302	28 June 1945	
304	5 August 1944	
306	15 August 1944	

307	4 September 1944	
312	19 July 1945	
314	2 June 1945	
316	9 June 1945	
318	31 July 1944	
321	21 July 1944	
323	10 August 1944	
325	29 August 1944	
326	8 June 1944	
327	12 June 1944	
328	17 July 1944	
331	7 July 1944	
332	17 September 1945	
333	25 August 1944	
334	2 November 1945	
British HATs		
56	11 September 1945	
58	Not recorded	
60	10 May 1946	
62	18 June 1946	
63	16 December 1945	
65	11 January 1947	
66	16 June 1947	
US HATs		
55	11 June 1945	
57	10 August 1945	
59	7 October 1945	
61	3 September 1945	
64	11 June 1945	
US OATs		
11	24 November 1944	
12	28 August 1944	
13	4 August 1944	Partly destroyed by fire at Newbury
14	23 November 1944	
15	31 July 1944	
17	9 August 1944	
27	22 June 1944	
31	10 July 1944	
33	18 August 1944	
36	28 August 1944	
37	16 November 1944	Brought into use 5 October

The eleven US OATs that had been used within Great Britain prior to D-Day were all withdrawn from use between late June and November 1944 in preparation for shipping to France. They were to join the twenty-six ambulance trains that were shipped across to be staffed by British and American medical personnel, as shown in the table below. The numbers may appear to be random and confusing, but when taken with the eleven used in Great Britain they create a sequence of thirty-seven ambulance trains numbered 11–47 that were known to have operated in Europe during Operation OVERLORD and the subsequent liberation of Europe. The War Office Ambulance Train Committee had agreed that forty-seven overseas ambulance trains would be made available in Europe by D-Day + 90.

Train Number	Rolling Stock	Staff	Date Shipped Overseas
25	LNER	British Army	31 August 1944
26	LNER	British Army	5 September 1944
28	LNER	British Army	25 September 1944
29	LNER	British Army	13 November 1944
30	LNER	British Army	14 November 1944
32	GWR	British Army	26 September 1944
34	GWR	British Army	2 October 1944
35	GWR	British Army	30 September 1944
42	LNER	British Army	3 November 1944
43	LNER	British Army	6 November 1944
45	GWR	British Army	10 November 1944
16	LMS	US Army	24 August 1944
18	LMS	US Army	29 September 1944
19	LMS	US Army	30 September 1944
20	LMS	US Army	23 September 1944
21	LMS	US Army	23 September 1944
22	LMS	US Army	1 October 1944
23	LMS	US Army	3 October 1944
24	LMS	US Army	5 October 1944
38	LMS	US Army	6 October 1944
39	LMS	US Army	8 October 1944
40	LMS	US Army	6 October 1944
41	LMS	US Army	13 October 1944
44	LNER	US Army	10 October 1944
46	GWR	US Army	10 October 1944
47	SR	US Army	12 October 1944

After the liberation of Belgium, which commenced on 2 September 1944, a Belgian ambulance train that consisted of a mixture of Belgian and British rolling stock

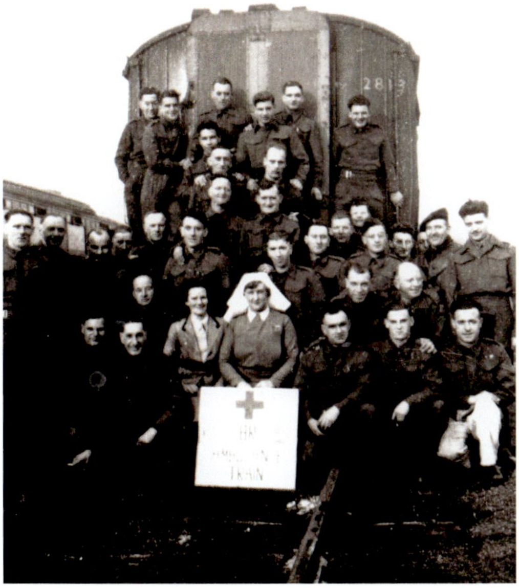

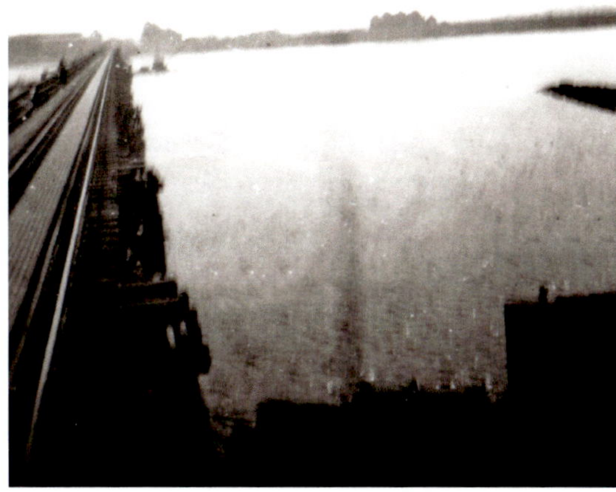

Above left: Staff of 45 (Overseas) Ambulance Train at Brussels, Christmas 1944. (A. Whitelock)

Above right: Photograph of the rail pontoon bridge across the River Rhine crossed by 45 (overseas) ambulance train. (A. Whitelock)

started to operate. The British stock had survived 'somewhere in France' since 1940. Trains were subsequently operated by Belgian and British RE train crew from a stabling point at Merelbeke on the outskirts of Ghent to Ostend and Brussels.[30]

An RAMC veteran who served on No. 45 (Overseas) Ambulance Train described operating in Belgium and Holland before crossing into Germany. This train was assembled from GWR rolling stock and was shipped overseas on 10 November 1944. Christmas 1944 found them in Brussels. The train was to cross into Germany over a rail pontoon bridge built across the River Rhine that was known as the Victory Bridge. In the reminiscences comment was made that: 'After a few weeks we were told that the train was moving up to a little station near Belsen Concentration Camp. None of us knew what to expect… The victims of man's inhumanity to man.'[31]

AIR EVACUATION RAILHEAD

During the planning for Operation OVERLORD the use of air evacuation of casualties, although in its relative infancy, was receiving increasing attention and therefore a rail/air interface needed to be considered. Four RAF stations were earmarked to receive casualties, with a planning figure of 600 per day. The four RAF stations were Down Ampney and Broadwell in Gloucestershire, Blakehill Farm in Wiltshire and Watchfield in Oxfordshire.

In May 1944 a decision was made that Shrivenham would be the railhead that would serve all four RAF stations and a dedicated ambulance train stabling facility would be constructed east of the Shrivenham GWR station. This would consist of two sidings with a 40-ft-wide road between them along with water points and storage facilities for ambulance train equipment. It is a testament to the hard work of GWR personnel and the government's Ministry of Works that the facility was completed in just five weeks and the first loaded ambulance train left on 22 June 1944.

Two trains were allocated to this Air Evacuation Railhead, namely No. 56 (Home) Ambulance Train and No. 321 Casualty Evacuation Train. By 21 July 1944, 321 CET had completed ten journeys and was replaced by No. 66 HAT. Records show that the proportion of lying to sitting casualties arriving by air was greater than anticipated, so in late August 1944 an extra ward coach, converted from an LNER bogie brake van, was added to each train.

The war diary of No. 66 HAT shows that it undertook many trips from Shrivenham to Birmingham and surrounding stations along with trips to Edinburgh in Scotland and Newport, Cardiff and Morriston in South Wales. Other destinations included Leicester, Nottingham, Derby and Worcester. Comments in the war diary clearly indicate that the earlier problems with the provision of stretcher bearers continued post D-Day and on one occasion medical students were drafted in to unload No. 66 HAT at Edinburgh.[32]

A peak was reached in August 1944, with three or four trains being despatched per day from Shrivenham, and thought was given to laying a third siding. Although planning took place, the scheme was abandoned in September 1944 as the casualty flows reduced to only needing two trains per day, and by the end of October 1944 the average was one train every two days.

AMBULANCE TRAINS IN OTHER THEATRES OF THE SECOND WORLD WAR

EAST AFRICA

The campaign in East Africa ran from June 1940 to November 1941 and was intertwined with the campaign in the Western Desert of North Africa as both campaigns aimed to safeguard the Suez Canal. Troops involved in the East Africa campaign were largely from the Union Defence Force of South Africa along with African colonial troops. The medical support to the campaign also initially came from the South African Medical Corps along with personnel from the Colonial Medical Services.[33] In September 1940 the Indian 5th Division arrived to support the campaign, bringing with it a range of medical units.[34]

The campaign encompassed Eritrea, Abyssinia (modern-day Ethiopia), Sudan, Uganda, Kenya and Somaliland. The railways within these countries were of several different gauges. The various operations within the campaign tended to have long lines of communication and rail evacuation was of value. However, the availability of rolling stock suitable for conversion was limited.

The ORBAT of the Sudan force in July 1941 included Nos 1, 2 and 3 (Sudan) Ambulance Trains and No. 2 (Egypt) Ambulance Train.[35] These four ambulance trains were all designed to carry seventy-six stretcher patients with the addition of extra coaches for sitting patients. In the period from September 1940 to August 1941 it is recorded that 22,155 patients were carried by rail, covering a total mileage of 70,428 miles.[36]

NORTH AFRICA

The North African Campaign ranged across Morocco, Algeria and Tunisia before encompassing Libya and Egypt and lasted from June 1942 until May 1943.[37] As will be expected, numerous detailed histories have been published covering the campaign and its many decisive operations.

During this period a range of railway gauges existed across the countries of North Africa and included standard-, metre- and narrow-gauge railways. This meant that the provision of any ambulance train capability relied on local rolling stock being available for conversion.

As part of the overall medical plan there were five French and four British ambulance trains operating in Algeria and Tunisia, along with empty freight wagons returning from the front line being utilised as necessary.[38] A contemporaneous account of ambulance train operating in Algeria and Tunisa was written by a medical officer who was there and he describes the four British standard-gauge trains.[39] One train was very poor and consisted of freight wagons and one or two non-corridor coaches. The other three were of much better standard and assembled from November 1942 and all had similar configurations, as shown in the table below.

Number	Vehicle Type	Converted to Role
1	Six-wheeled 1st /2nd class coach	Guard and spare engine crew accommodation
1	Six-wheeled van	Kitchen and dispensary
1	Six-wheeled 1st/2nd class corridor coach	Staff accommodation
2	Six-wheeled 1st/2nd class corridor coach	72 sitting patients each
2	Mail van	30 lying patients each
1	Luggage van	30 lying patients
1	Six-wheeled corridor coach	Offices, MOs' and NOs' accommodation

These three trains were approximately 240 tons of unladen weight each. They had a capacity of ninety lying and 172 sitting patients managed by a staff of thirty. They were stabled at Souk Ahras in Algeria and evacuated patients on a regular basis to Algiers with a journey time of some twenty-two hours.[40]

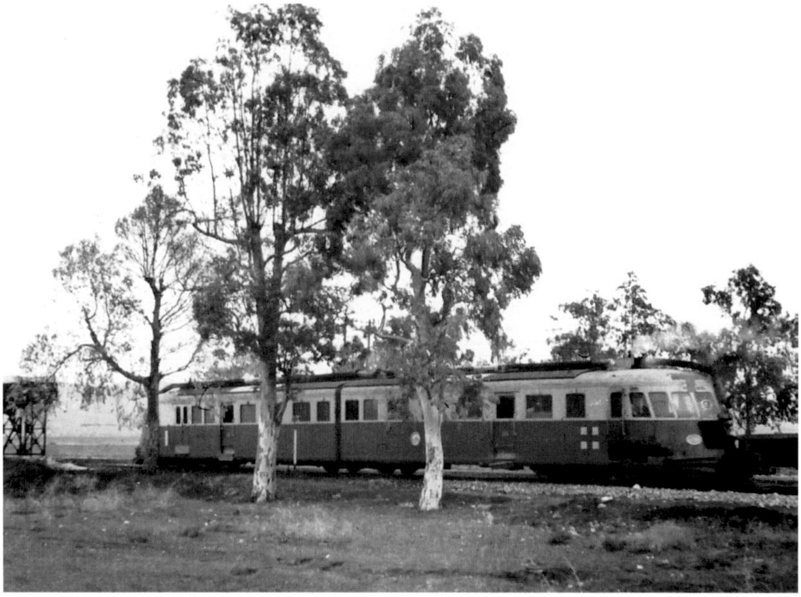

Diesel railcars used in Tunisia and Algeria during the North African Campaign. (© Imperial War Museum NA506)

Mention should also be made of six Michelin diesel railcars coupled in pairs that were locally sourced and were converted to carry twenty-one lying and twenty-four sitting patients. They mainly operated between Souk-el-Khems and Souk Ahras. After the fall of Tunis these railcars continued to run regular services between Tunis and Souk-Ahras.[41] There was also some metre-gauge ambulance train activity between Tebesso and Constantine in Algeria.[42]

ITALY

The Italian Campaign commenced with the invasion of Sicily in July 1943 that led to the fall of the fascist Italian regime led by Mussolini. The campaign is often also referred to as the Liberation of Italy as, even with the fall of the fascists, Italy had been occupied by German forces from September 1943. The troops who fought in the Italian Campaign are often referred to as one of the Second World War's 'Forgotten Armies', yet their hard-fought battles resulted in many casualties. After Sicily, the Allies landed on mainland Italy at Salerno and Taranto. There followed an advance northwards to liberate the whole of Italy.[43]

In the medical planning for the invasion of the Italian mainland the general plan was to evacuate casualties to North Africa and the Middle East, with air evacuation being the preferred option. Casualties were to be landed at Tunis in Tunisia, Bône (modern-day Annaba) and Philippeville (modern-day Skikda), both in Algeria. Of particular interest, the plan refers to the availability of what are referred to as hospital trains in North Africa with one a day running from Tunis to Constantine and Philippeville and two trains per week running from Constantine and Philippeville to Algiers.[44]

The first reference to ambulance trains operating on the Italian mainland appears to be in early October 1943 when locally converted stock commenced a service between Bari on the east coast to Taranto, a distance of approximately 100 km.[45] With the advance northwards, the reach of ambulance trains also increased and by December 1943 an evacuation route was established southwards along the coast from Termoli to Bari. Records show that four trains ran on the route but no details as to their composition or staffing have survived. It is interesting that after two trains were removed, one damaged beyond use and the other redeployed elsewhere, overcrowding of the CCSs around Termoli resulted. This clearly showed the importance of rail evacuation.[46]

With the advance northwards the four battles fought around Monte Cassino between January and May 1944 are considered the hardest fought of the whole war. Nearly a quarter of a million troops drawn from six continents were involved. The large number of casualties from Cassino were evacuated south by road to Cancello, from where ambulance trains ran to Bari on the east coast and then southwards to Taranto.[47] Extremely severe weather in early 1944 damaged infrastructure and hampered ambulance train operating.

After the fall of Rome on 5 June 1944 there was a consolidation of the evacuation effort as the Allies advanced northwards. In August 1944 it is recorded that ambulance train railheads were established at Aresso, Assisi and Lesi, with evacuation routes south to Rome and Naples. At this time there was also the opportunity to separate cases by nationality and route them to their own national facilities. British casualties were evacuated down the west coast of Italy whilst New Zealand, Indian and South African casualties were moved to the east coast for onward evacuation by sea.

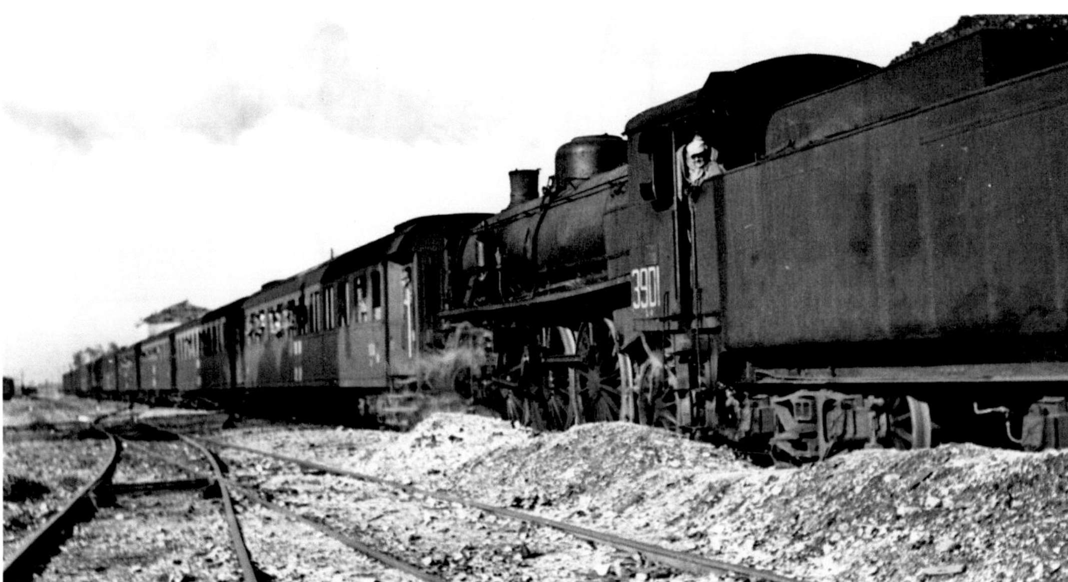

A US ambulance train leaves for Naples in February 1944 following the Battle of Cassino. (ACME)

In July and August 1944 there was a re-organisation of Allied ambulance trains, although what prompted this is not clear. Nos 1 (Egyptian), 2, 6, 70 and 71 Ambulance Trains were disbanded and reformed as 77, 78, 79 and 80 Ambulance Trains. To these were added 20, 21 and 22 (North African) Ambulance Trains along with No. 12 (Indian) Ambulance Train, making a total of eight trains. The reference to an Indian ambulance train serves as a reminder that other Allies also provided ambulance trains. Although still referred to as hospital trains, in July 1943 the No. 66 (US) Hospital Train commenced operating within Italy followed in November 1943 by No. 41 (US) Hospital Train.

Following the Allies' advance northward, German forces in Italy finally capitulated on 2 May 1945.

GREECE

A small Commonwealth expeditionary force comprising Australian, New Zealand and British forces was sent to Greece after Italy attacked Greece in October 1940. The campaign only lasted from 6 to 28 April 1941. The medical ORBAT for the campaign lists three ambulance trains, although it is far from clear whether these trains ever became fully operational. Staff and equipment to create two trains had been sent from Egypt, but the locally available rolling stock was reported as being of very poor quality.

One train, designated No. 2 Ambulance Train, was improvised and a second train obtained on loan from Greece. The latter was subsequently split to create 1A and 1B Ambulance Trains staffed by a mix of Greek and British personnel. The No. 2 Ambulance Train was entirely staffed by British personnel. All these three trains were based at Athens.[48]

BURMA AND INDIA

The Burma Campaign was part of the wider South East Asia theatre of the Second World War and, like all major campaigns, many detailed histories have been published. The campaign involved British and Commonwealth forces against the invading forces of Japan who landed in Burma in January 1942. Burma had ceased to be a province of India in 1937 and became politically independent, although only had a degree of self-government. The defence of Burma had remained the responsibility of the British governor. It is fair to say that Burma was as good as defenceless against the strength of Japan. The Burma Campaign is usually divided into four phases. Firstly, Japan invaded Burma leading to the expulsion of British, Indian and Chinese forces in 1942. There were then various failed Allied offensive incursions into Burma from India between late 1942 and early 1944 to attempt to dislodge the Japanese forces. Japan then attempted to invade India in 1944, followed by the final phase involving the Allied liberation of Burma between late

1944 and mid-1945. The geography and terrain of the region, weather and disease prevalence were all to influence the various operations.

As with so many overseas campaigns, details about ambulance train activity, where it occurred, is very sketchy. It is recorded in one source that fourteen ambulance trains and three individual ambulance coaches operated on Burma's metre-gauge network during the campaign.[49] In another source eleven individual ambulance trains are recorded.[50]

With the outbreak of war in Europe, the Burma Army was expanded and Indian troops also moved into Burma in early 1941. There was an initial medical ORBAT to meet the perceived need of two field ambulances, two casualty clearing stations, two general hospitals, two field hygiene sections, two ambulance trains and two motor ambulance sections.[51] There was, however, a significant shortfall of medical officers and nurses to staff all these units. The two ambulance trains entered service in December 1941 having been converted from first- and second-class Burma Railway metre-gauge carriages and were identified as Nos 1 and 2 (Burma) Ambulance Trains. It is known that stretchers had to be loaded through windows and that the stock was non-corridor. Each train carried 100 lying or 200 sitting patients. It is recorded that they 'were stocked with fourteen days' rations and with plenty of medical comforts'.[52]

A third ambulance train was converted at Mandalay and records show that in just one week it moved 1,050 patients from Rangoon to Prome. A fourth train was also procured but it never entered service as the evacuation of Rangoon intervened in the face of the Japanese advance.[53]

As the Japanese forces advanced and the Allies withdrew towards the India and China borders, ambulance trains and river steamers were used to evacuate hospitals throughout the country. One example describes the use of an ambulance train with additional coaches carrying a full load of patients along with the staff from No. 2 Burma General Hospital, a district laboratory and a dental centre some 360 miles from Maymyo to Myitkyino, from where the staff and patients were all evacuated by air into India.[54]

Once the final phase of the campaign, the Allied liberation of Burma, was underway ambulance trains are recorded again in the medical ORBAT. They all appear to be Indian ambulance trains and their Indian bases are recorded. No. 14 (Indian) Ambulance Train was based in Dibrugarh in north-east India, Nos 17 and 19 (Indian) Ambulance Trains are recorded at Manipur Road and Nos 20, 21, 22 and 29 (Indian) Ambulance Trains all operated out of Chittagong, which is in modern-day Bangladesh, and ran south into Burma.

5

Post-Second World War

Although many of the ambulance trains used in Europe during the Second World War were decommissioned, the British Army continued to use ambulance trains to move sick and injured through the British corridor of occupied Europe on their journey home.

A most unusual item of rolling stock was British Army Railcar No. 1. This was an eight-wheeled Belgian State Railways railcar converted in 1945 to take twenty-seven stretchers in three tiers. This railcar, along with a second one, only operated between 1945 and 1947.

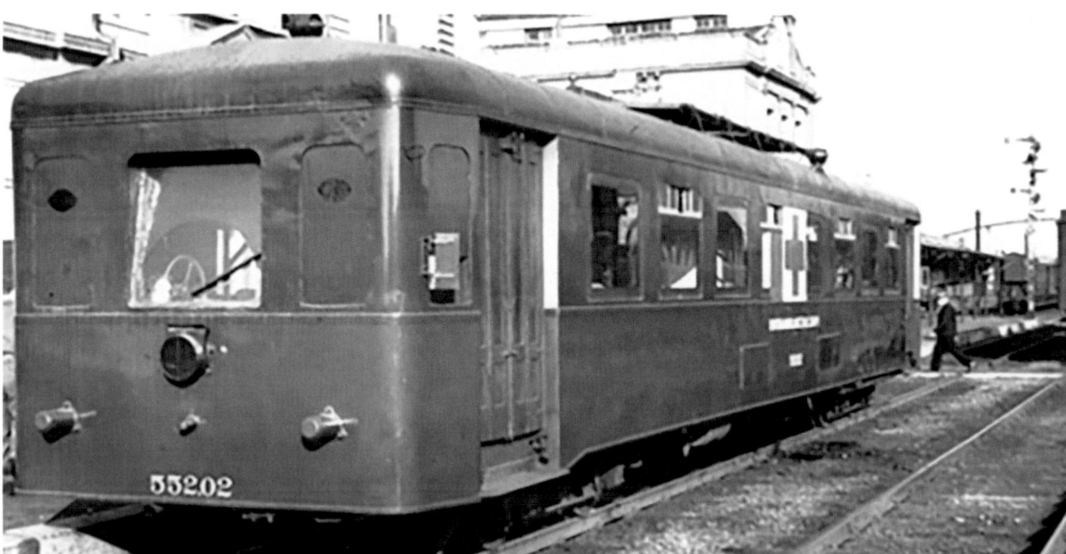

British Army Railcar No. 1 at Renaix (now Ronse) on 17 February 1945. (© Imperial War Museum B14689)

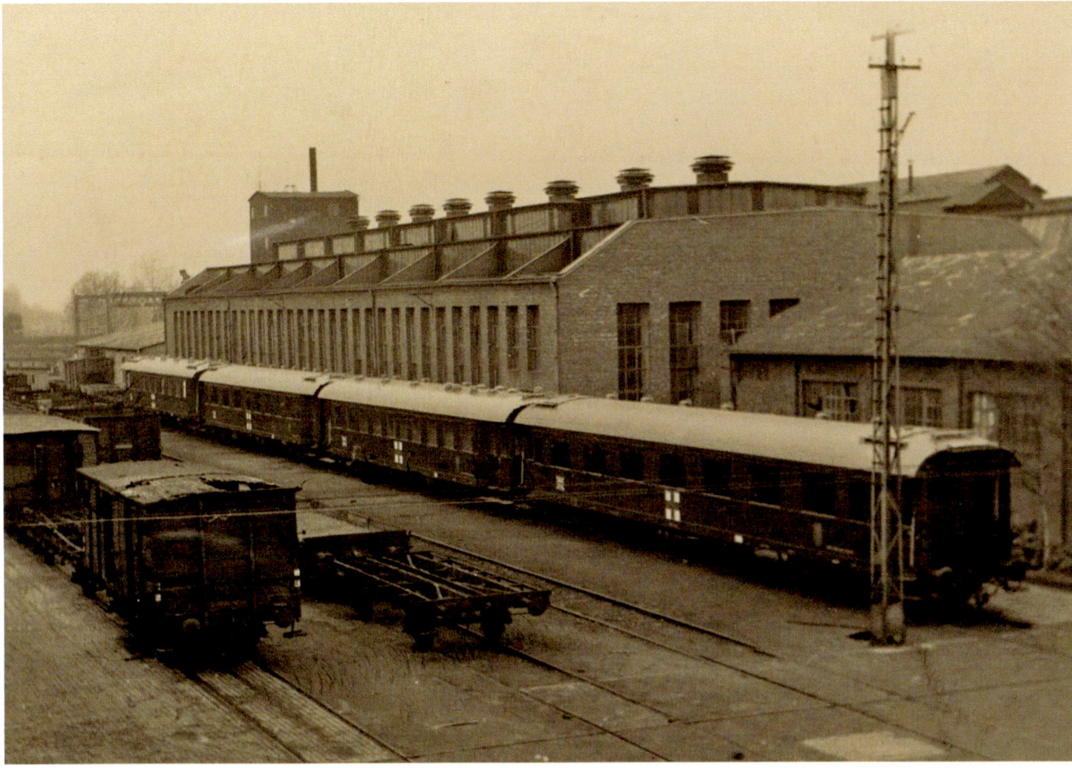

Four of the coaches that would form part of British Army Ambulance Train No. 1 awaiting handover at *Waggonfabrik Uerdingen AG* in 1946. (Museum of Military Medicine. Ref: RAMC/1240)

The railcars operated a feeder service around Brussels and carried patients to join British Army Ambulance Train No. 1, that ran the length of the British zone transporting sick and injured on the first stage of their journey home. This immediate post-war ambulance train was commissioned by the Royal Engineers Branch of HQ BAOR and built between September and December 1946 by two German railway workshops, *Waggenfabrik Uerdingen AG* and *Düsseldorfer Waggonfabrik AG*. This was a sixteen-coach train and its nine ward coaches carried 250 patients. This train was routed through the British zone from Osnabrück via Wuppertal, Munster and Hannover to Hamburg. Here the patients were transferred to the HS *El Nil* for the journey across the English Channel.

British Army Ambulance Train No. 1 was commanded by a major RAMC and staffed by one other RAMC officer, two nursing sisters, a warrant officer class 2 and thirty-three other ranks. The nursing sisters who would have initially been QAIMNS became the QARANC in 1949. This train continued to run through the British corridor until air trooping and air evacuation of casualties took over in the early 1960s.

With the day-to-day evacuation of casualties from BAOR being undertaken by the scheduled services of British Army Ambulance Train No. 1, plans were drawn up to acquire and convert fourteen ex-DR buffet coaches into open-ward coaches. These would be the nucleus of an ambulance train capability within BAOR ready for any future conflict in Europe that would last throughout the Cold War.

Turning back to England at the end of hostilities, in 1945 the individual ambulance cars referred to earlier were all returned to Netley Hospital. Little use seems to have been made of them and they were eventually transferred to the Longmoor Military Railway in 1954/55.[1] It is not known how many were retained as a usable ambulance capability as many were incorporated in other roles. Four of them were known to have been retained in an ambulance role and were made available to British Railways for the Lourdes pilgrimage traffic.

In 1958 four SR Maunsell coaches were converted to an ambulance role to replace those of the ex-LSWR dining saloons that were still in that role. These four had 'AMBULANCE CAR' on the sides of the green-liveried coaches. This stock was also rarely used but made available to British Railways, on a few occasions, to support Lourdes pilgrimage traffic.

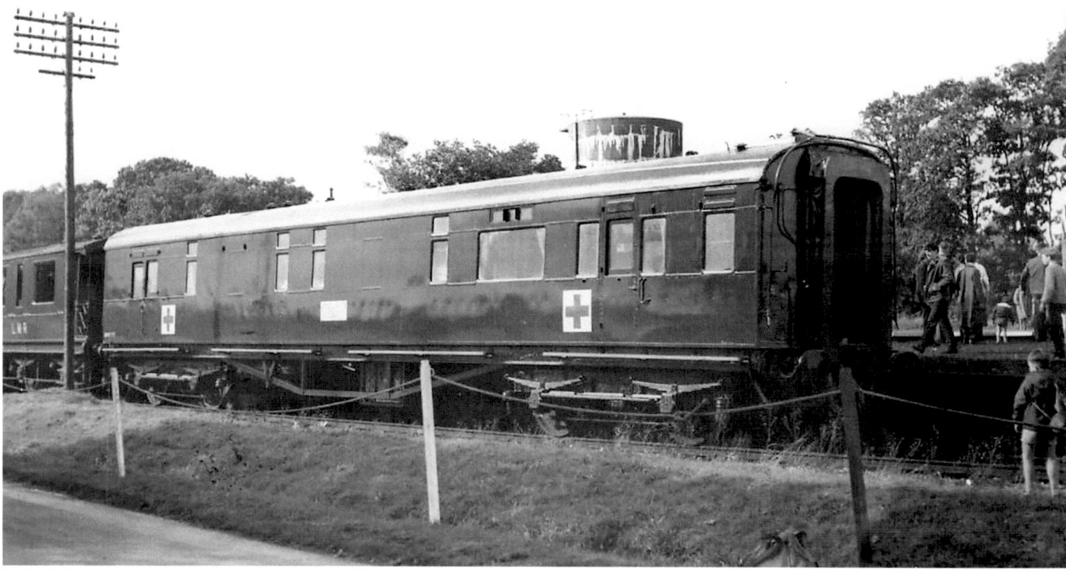

Ambulance coach 777 (S7921S) at the Longmoor Military Railway Open Day, 28 September 1968. (George M. Moon)

6
Korean War

The Korean War took place between 25 June 1950 and 27 July 1953 between North Korea, backed by China and the Soviet Union, and South Korea, supported by sixteen countries from the United Nations. In addition, five other countries provided non-combatant personnel.[1] Some 18,000 British troops deployed to Korea in support of the United Nations force, with 1,106 killed in action.

At the start of the Korean War there were no ambulance trains and very few medical facilities. Early improvised rail transport saw stretchers laid across the wooden seats of local rolling stock. After a rather haphazard beginning plans were made for properly converted rolling stock to be shipped to Korea from the United States. The first dedicated hospital train rolling stock arrived from the USA in November 1950. These were 84-ft-long (26-m) bogie coaches built in 1944 and 1945 for use within continental USA that had been in storage since the end of the Second World War.[2] By the end of 1951 all hospital trains had been amalgamated into a single US Army unit, the 8138th Army Unit hospital trains.

Within this unit all available rolling stock was divided into eight trains numbered 101–108 hospital trains. These were seven-coach trains including kitchen and pharmacy coaches. All the trains were based at Pusan Harbour and ran continuously to and from the front using separate dedicated north and south routings.[3] These trains operated under the auspices of the United Nations with US Army crew, so are outside the scope of this work.

Although not actually within Korea itself, mention must be made of British involvement operating ambulance train coaches attached to scheduled Japanese trains within Japan during the war and immediately after the cessation of hostilities. The author was given some personal notes by an RAMC veteran who had served on these coaches between August 1953 and September 1954. The usual arrangement was of one or two coaches converted for stretchers and a coach for walking casualties staffed by one or two QARANC sisters, two male RAMC orderlies and two Japanese Railway employees.[4]

These British-operated ambulance coaches were utilised to and from the United National Air Base at Iwakumi and the British Commonwealth General Hospital at Kure. Casualties were flown out of Korea to Japan and also from Japan back to the UK. The layout of the rolling stock that was used was described by a QARANC nursing sister in a memoire of her service during the Korean War.[5] The coaches had centre double doors and on one side was a ward area of sixteen bunks in two tiers for lying patients and to the other side an office, treatment room and kitchen.

The Korean War was a costly conflict that is often referred to as another 'Forgotten War'. There were 170,927 dead and 32,585 declared missing amongst the UN forces, along with an estimate of somewhere between 398,000 and 926,000 killed amongst North Korean and Chinese forces. Total wounded have been estimated at between 500,000 and 700,000 across both sides. Total civilian dead have also been estimated at 2 to 3 million.[6] Although an Armistice was signed on 27 July 1953, the war has never officially ended. The Armistice was signed by the USA representing the United Nations, the Korean People's Army and the China People's Volunteer Army. However, South Korea refused to sign.

The Korean War should not be forgotten in the history of ambulance trains operating as rail was effectively used largely due to the poor condition of Korean roads. Air evacuation was also rapidly developing but rail was needed to deliver casualties to safe airheads for onward evacuation.

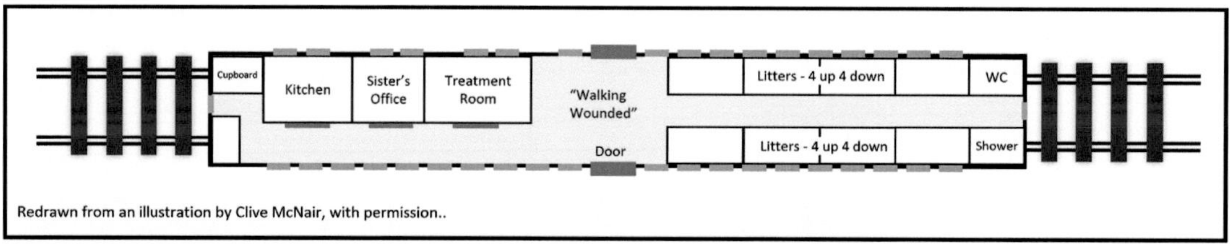

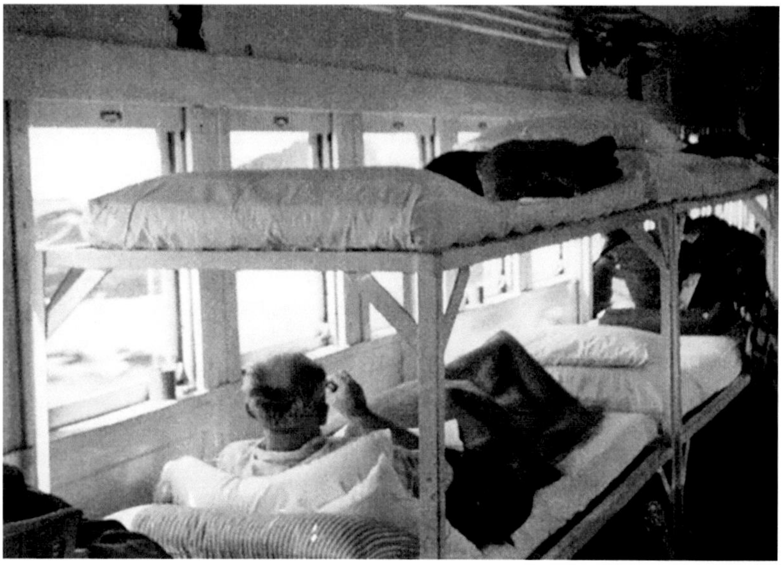

Above: Diagrammatic layout of an ambulance coach as used by the British in Japan during and after the Korean War. (Redrawn with permission from an illustration by Clive McNair)

Left: The interior of one of the ambulance coaches used in Japan. (E. J. McNair)

7
Cold War

The Cold War lasted from 1947 to 1991 and was a period of political tension between the United States of America along with its Western Bloc Allies and the Soviet Union with its Eastern Bloc Allies. Although no actual fighting occurred between the two superpowers, there were periods of heightened tension with regional conflicts in Korea and the Middle East. Ever present was the arms race and the fear of nuclear annihilation. Integral to the Cold War was the North Atlantic Treaty Organisation (NATO) and within that the British Army of the Rhine (BAOR).

NATO AND BAOR

NATO is an intergovernmental military alliance of thirty-two member states. Originally formed by just twelve countries on 4 April 1949, following the end of the Second World War, it has its HQ in Brussels in Belgium.[1] BAOR was considered to be the first line of British defence through its contribution to NATO. It is worth remembering that there have been two British Armies of the Rhine. The first BAOR was established in May 1919 to oversee the British occupation of the Rhineland following the end of the First World War. That BAOR remained in Germany until 1929.

The second BAOR was established within West Germany, following the end of the Second World War. Initially the British Liberation Army that had previously landed on the beaches of Normandy was re-designated the 21st Army Group, which then became BAOR on 25 August 1945. Historically, the British Army had been used to gaining and garrisoning lands around the world for the empire, but in terms of Europe expeditionary forces had been sent in wartime. BAOR was to be very different and evolved into a major military force permanently stationed in Germany. This was not just the soldiers but their wives and families along with their schools, shops, cinemas and hospitals. Despite this apparent normality, BAOR had to be ready to go to war at a moment's notice.[2, 3]

Throughout the following years BAOR underwent many reorganisations to meet the perceived and ever-changing threats as the Cold War evolved.[4] The stylised map below illustrates the 1st British Corps Area of responsibility within NATO which was commonly referred to as 'the Corridor'. It was within this Corps area that the British Army ambulance trains trained and operated in preparation for any future conflict in Europe. Often referred to as the 'NATO layer cake', various member countries had different geographical areas of military responsibility.

In addition to the fact that West Germany was divided into NATO military areas of responsibility the city of Berlin was divided between the east and west, with West Berlin consisting of French, British and American sectors and East Berlin being

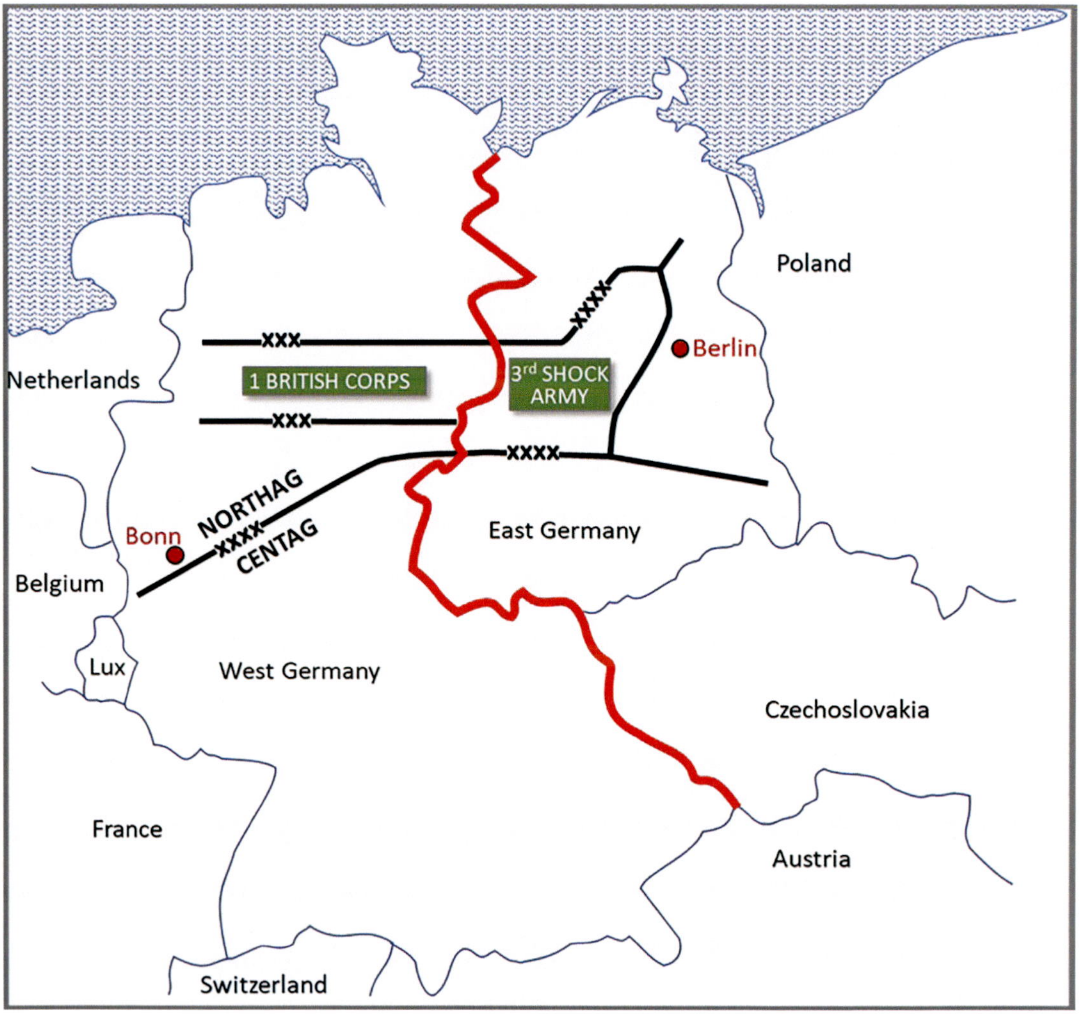

A stylised map of Germany during the Cold War illustrating the 1st British Corps area of responsibility commonly referred to as 'the Corridor'. (Drawn by Sally Finlayson)

under Soviet control. The 28½ miles of the Berlin Wall divided the Allied sectors from the Soviet east. Sitting as it did within East Germany, there was also a 70-mile border around the three Allied sectors and the rest of East Germany. To complete this very brief historical overview, the Berlin Wall was eventually demolished in November 1989 and the demise of the Soviet Union followed in 1992. BAOR was disbanded on 28 October 1994, with the remaining British forces redesignated British Forces Germany but still firmly committed to NATO.

AMBULANCE TRAIN OPERATING IN BAOR

Prior to 1985 the British Army operated a number of individual ambulance train staffs, but they were rarely exercised. An MoD re-organisation in 1985 created the Ambulance Train Squadron RAMC(V), an AMS TA Specialist Unit. This consisted of ten trains numbered 330–39 Ambulance Trains RAMC(V). Based in the UK, the squadron was committed to BAOR on mobilisation. One of the trains was a Continental TA unit. Raised in 1984, the Continental TA consisted of a range of units based within BAOR and staffed by eligible personnel who were resident within mainland Europe. 335 (BAOR) Ambulance Train RAMC(V) was part of the Ambulance Train Squadron but based in Mönchengladbach in BAOR.

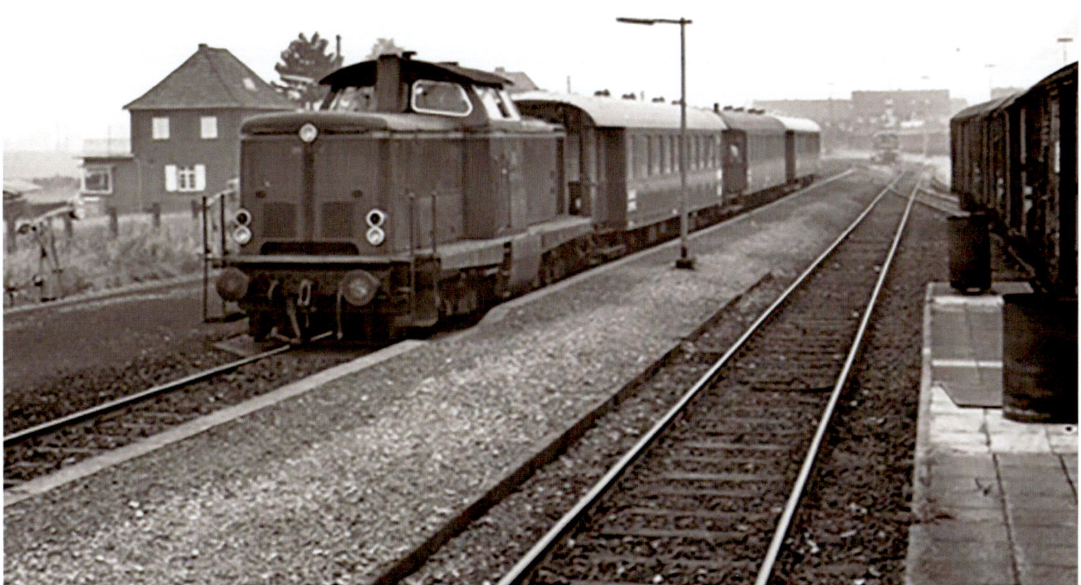

A 1972 ambulance train exercise 'somewhere in BAOR'.

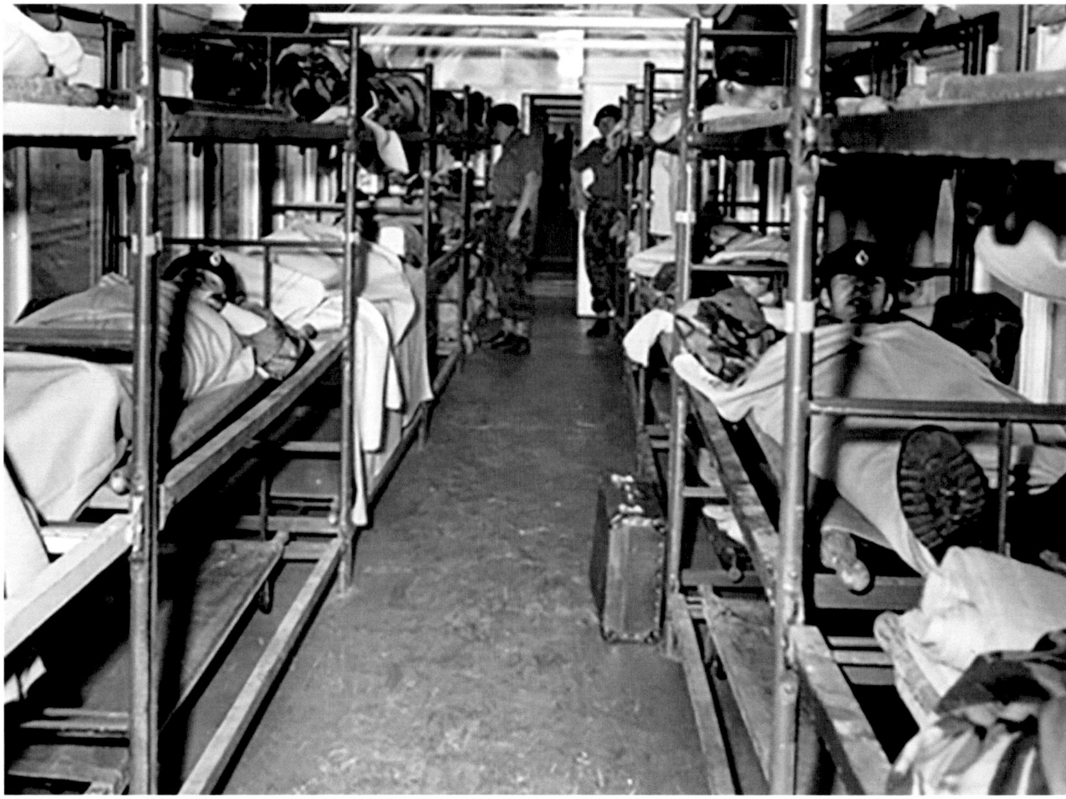

Interior of the post-war ex-DR rolling stock on exercise in BAOR in 1972.

Each train had a staff of six officers and thirty-three ORs, giving a squadron total of sixty officers and 330 ORs. There would be an increase of fifteen per train at war establishment.

Between 1980 and 1994 trains were operated every year in support of medical formation and larger corps exercises. Most of the AMS and wider TA only exercised in BAOR once every three years but as the ambulance trains were of Continental-gauge stock and based in BAOR the Ambulance Train Squadron deployed to Germany every year. Usually, two trains were exercised each year, with three deployed simultaneously on Exercise FOLDING BED 88. These regular exercises ensured that staff developed considerable expertise in operating ambulance trains.

It is worthy of mention that both the German Army (Bundeswehr) and the Dutch Army had ambulance train capability during the Cold War years, both staffed by their respective reserve armies. They were, however, not exercised to anywhere near the same extent as the British Army trains.

Ambulance trains were an integrated part of the whole casualty evacuation system through which casualties would have been moved back to the Channel Ports. Ambulance trains were planned to run in two loops. A short-haul loop was run from the field hospitals of the Forward Surgical Complex (FSC) within the Forward Combat Zone (FCZ) back to the general hospitals in the Rear Combat Zone (RCZ).

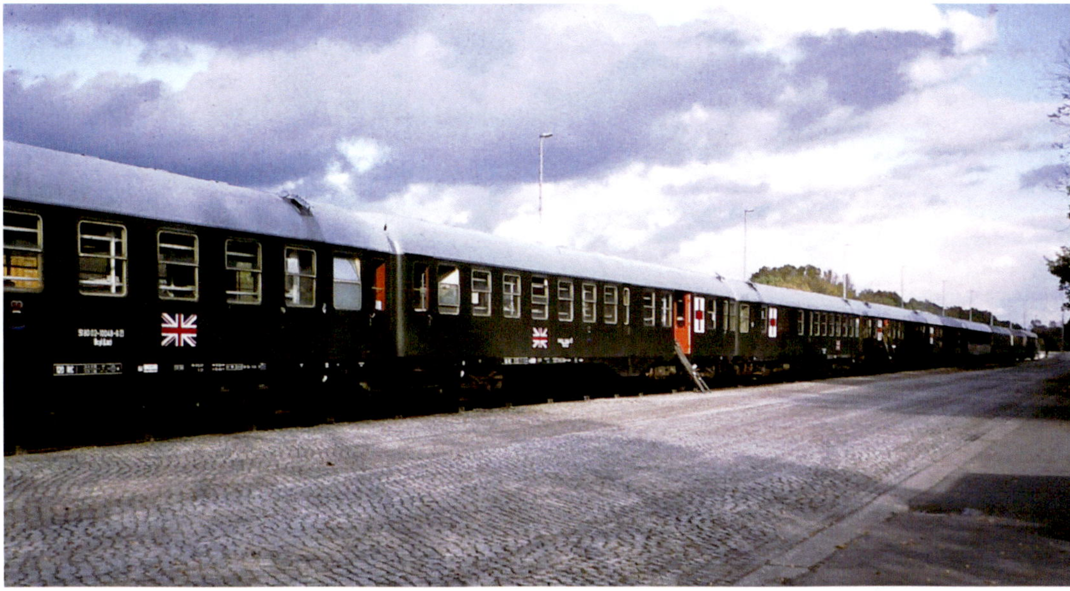

One of two ambulance trains deployed on Exercise FLYING SCOT 93 at Hohne.

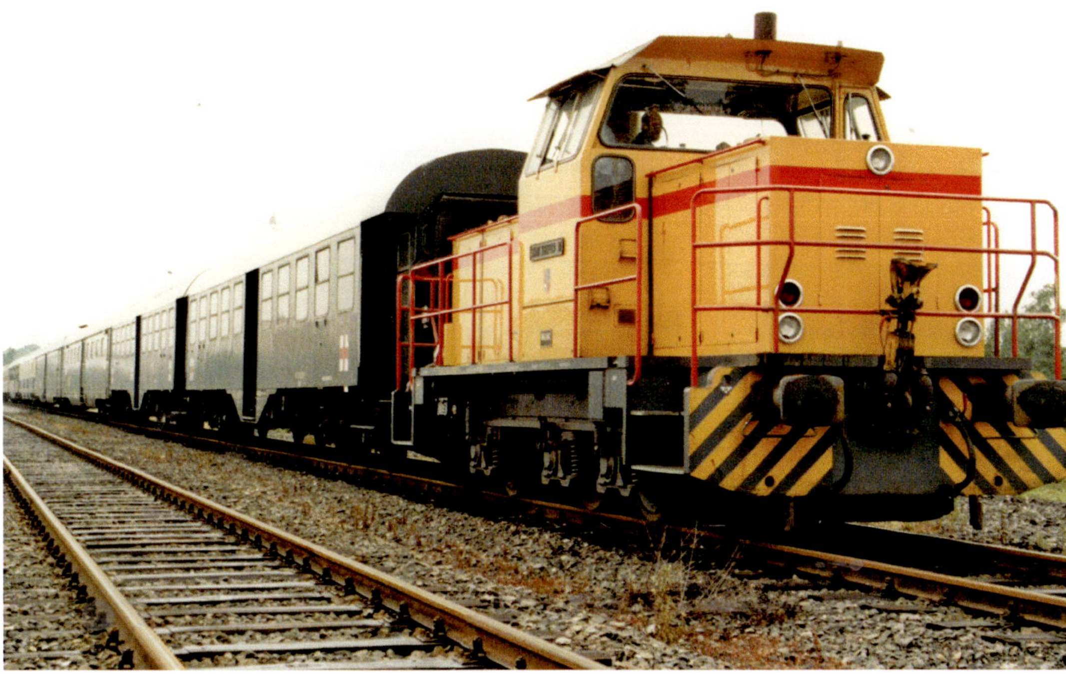

One of two ambulance trains deployed on Exercise FOLDING BED 89 approaching Krefeld Linn.

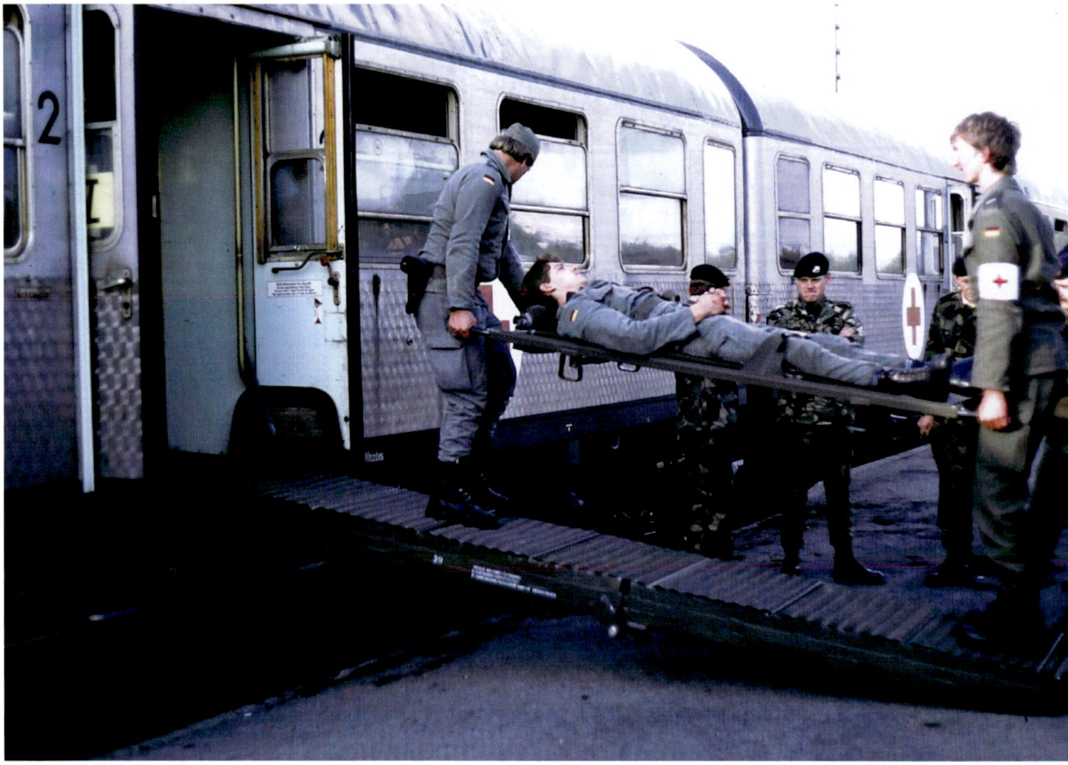

A Bundeswehr ambulance train in 1985.

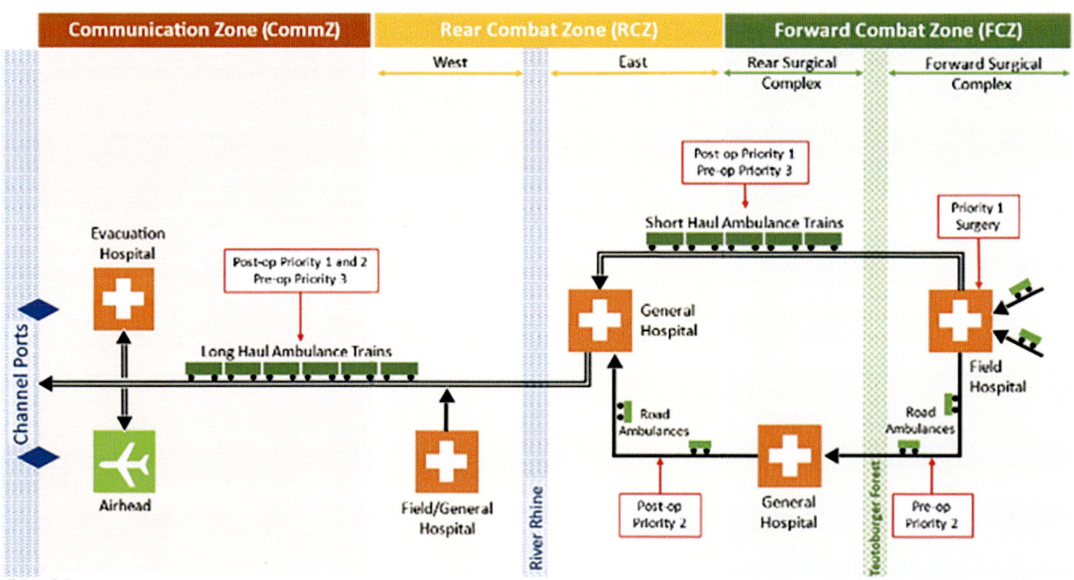

A schematic representation of the chain of evacuation for casualties within BAOR during the Cold War. (Drawn by Sally Finlayson)

There were then long-haul trains that ran back from the RCZ to the evacuation or port hospitals and airheads of the Communications Zone (Comm Z) or direct to the Channel Ports. The crossings of the Channel would have been undertaken with ships under RN control taken up from trade (STUFT) such as the Ro-Ro ferries regularly crossing the Channel.

The Ambulance Train Squadron RAMC(V) was reorganised in 1994 to become the Ambulance Train Group RAMC(V), with its ten trains reduced to four. The establishment of each train was increased in this re-organisation to fifteen officers and forty-one ORs. The group was to be short-lived, being disbanded in 1995 as part of the drawdown of BAOR.

AMBULANCE TRAIN ROLLING STOCK

Mention was made earlier of a small amount of rolling stock was converted for ambulance train purposes after the Second World War and retained within BAOR. As the Cold War progressed three different types of rolling stock have been incorporated into the British Army ambulance train fleet, and each will be described below.

EX-US ARMY REPARATION STOCK DESIGNATED BYMK

A fleet of purpose-built ambulance stock was constructed in 1952 under a reparation agreement for the US Army. Linke-Hofmann-Busch of Salzgitter built sixty-five vehicles as dual-purpose troop sleeping and ambulance coaches for use by the US Army Transportation Corps (USATC). They were amongst a number of different types of rail vehicles built for the USATC during the period 1952–56 which included sleeping, personnel and kitchen diners along with utility coaches that provided power for heating and light.

The sixty-five ward coaches entered service with the USATC in March 1953. All of the ward coaches were 26.4 m long, 2.83 m wide, 4.05 m high and each had an unladen weight of 44.5 tonnes.

In October 1974, thirty-two of the ambulance ward coaches, three kitchen diners and a staff coach were transferred to the British Army. All of these vehicles had been operated in ambulance train formations by the USATC and the US Army Medical Department. Ownership of the vehicles was recorded in the individual rolling stock records as being transferred from the USA Rail Maintenance Group to UK HQ BAOR.

The thirty-two ward coaches carried the DB rolling stock designation code *Bymk* and each had forty-two berths per coach. They were intended for the long-haul runs from the RCZ to the Comm Z. The casualties were transferred from their stretchers to bunks for a more comfortable ride in view of the length of the journey. This required stretchers to be carried on the train or a further supply made available at the rear railhead to facilitate unloading.

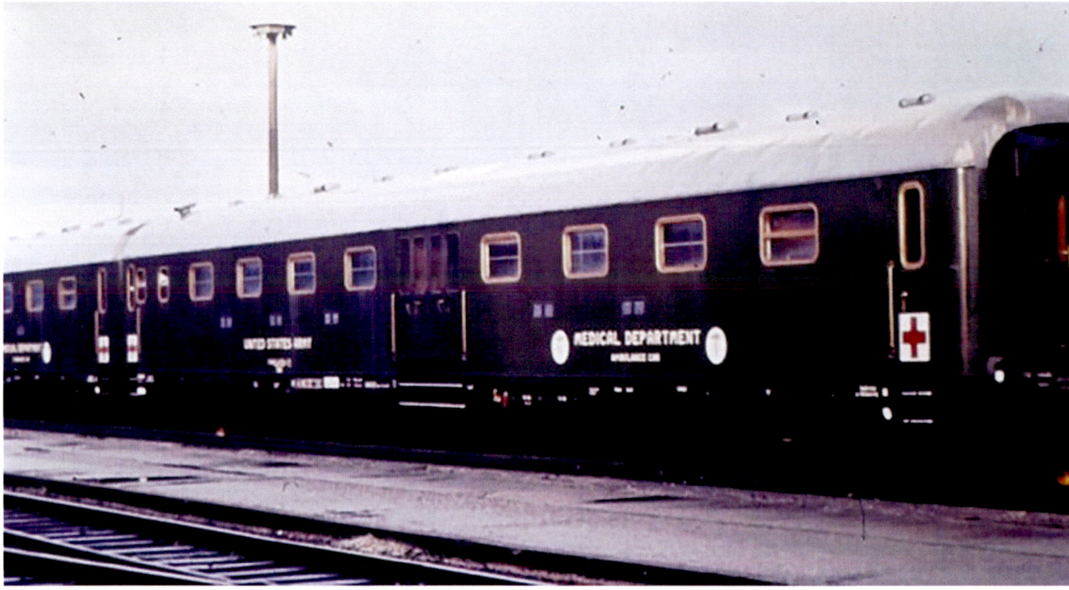

A *Bymk* ward coach in original US Army Medical Department livery.

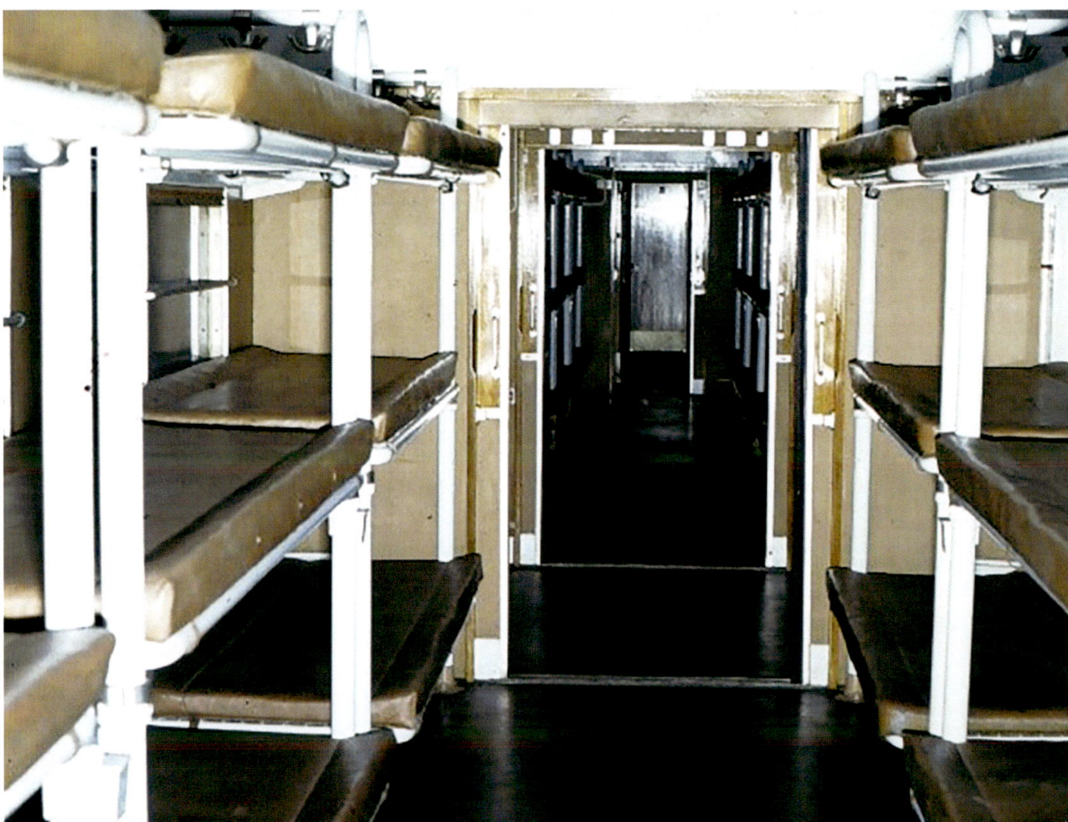

The interior of a *Bymk* ward coach.

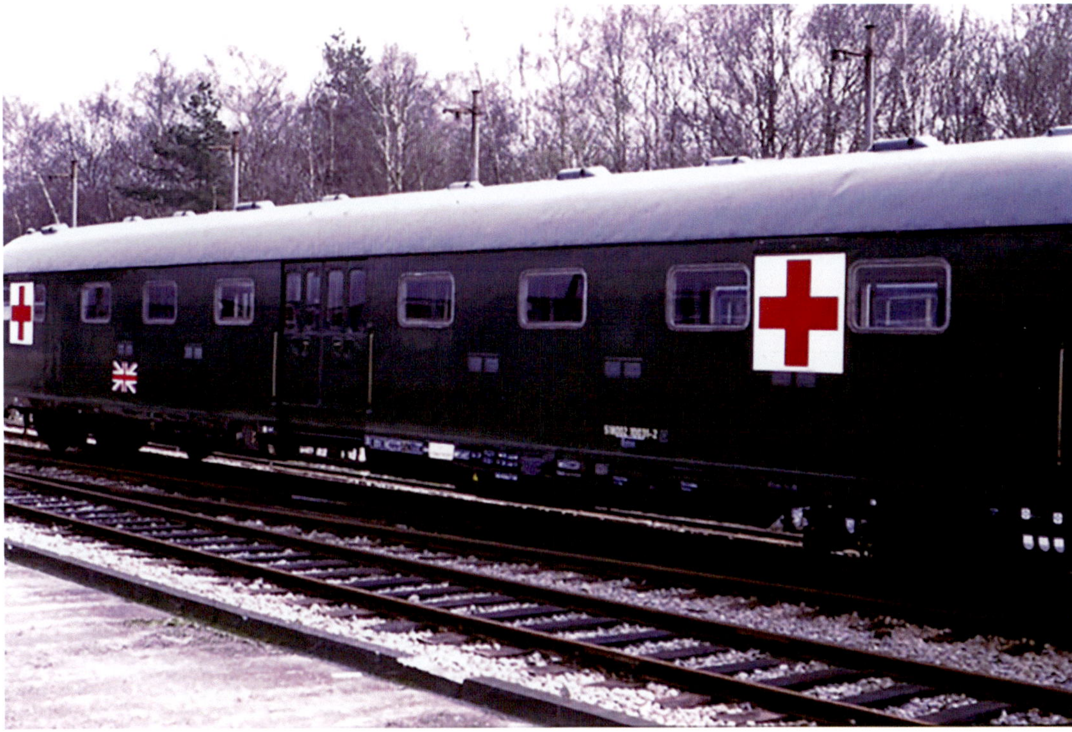

The prototype refurbished *Bymk* ward coach at 79 Railway Squadron RCT in 1988.

In 1988 an upgrade and refurbishment programme was started for the *Bymk* fleet. The plan was that some five or six coaches per year would be upgraded with a number of significant features. These were a complete electrical overhaul along with the provision of illuminated external Red Cross emblems in accordance with the Geneva Convention. The provision of a water carriage pack in each coach would reduce the number of berths to forty-one per coach. The installation of internal communications throughout a train was to be provided along with external communication via the wider DB network. Finally, each coach would be repainted.

This refurbishment was undertaken against the background that these coaches were already over thirty years old. The programme was discontinued when a decision was made to purchase some replacement stock from the DB and all the *Bymk* stock was retired. Some of the fleet continued to serve as staff accommodation on exercises and during other military tasks.

EX-DB ROLLING STOCK DESIGNATED BYG

In 1977–78 the British Army obtained twelve ex-DB passenger coaches carrying the DB designation *Byg*. These originally dated from 1957 and were converted to take thirty stretchers on frames.

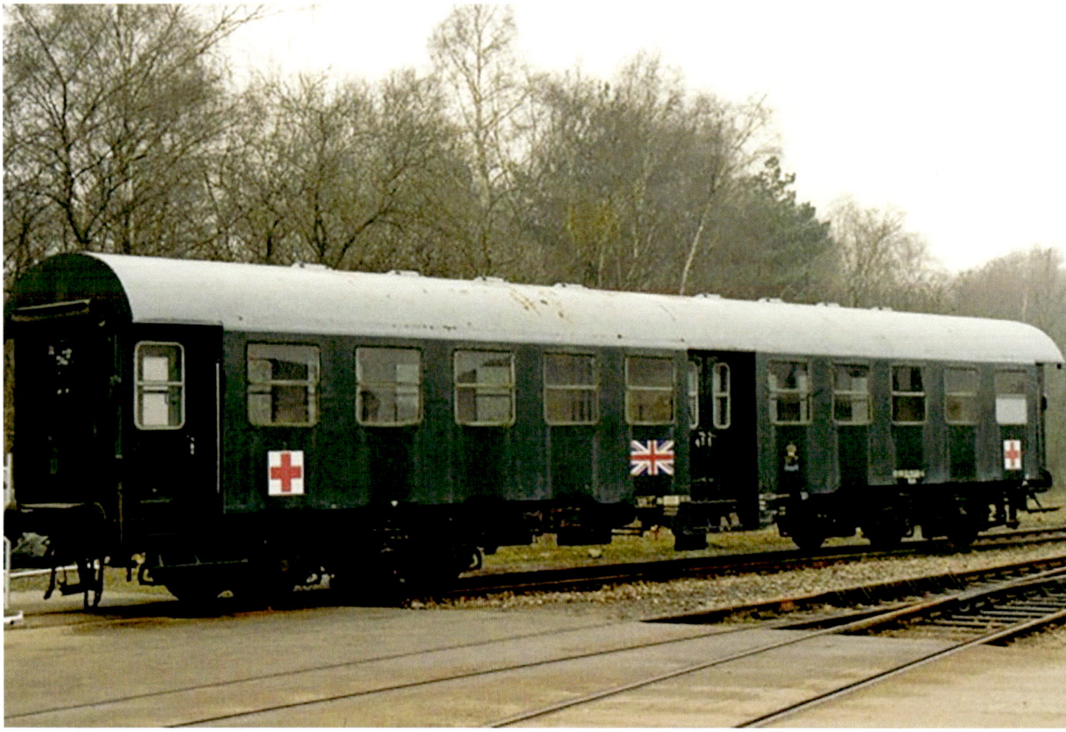

A *Byg* ward coach at 79 Railway Squadron RCT.

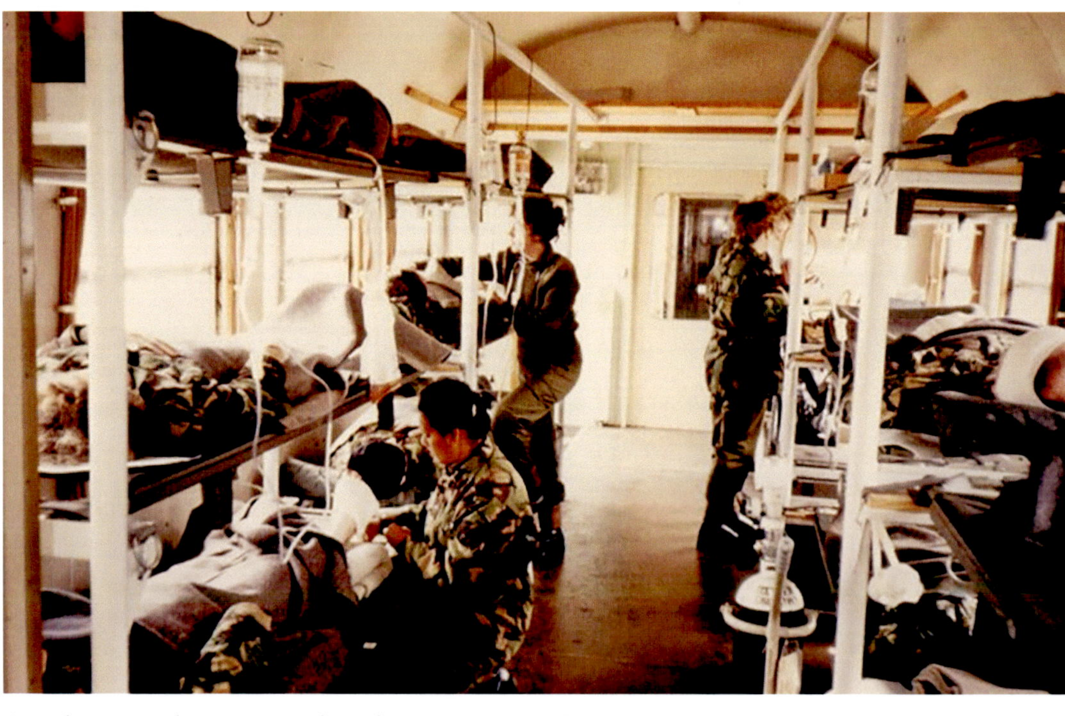

Casualty care within a *Byg* ward coach on Exercise FOLDING BED 87.

EX-DB ROLLING STOCK DESIGNATED BCYL (LAZ)

In 1990 delivery started of a number of replacement coaches that effectively stopped the *Bymk* refurbishment programme. These coaches originally dated from 1954 and came directly from revenue earning on the DB network. They were converted in the British Army REME Workshops at Wetter in West Germany to take forty stretchers per coach.

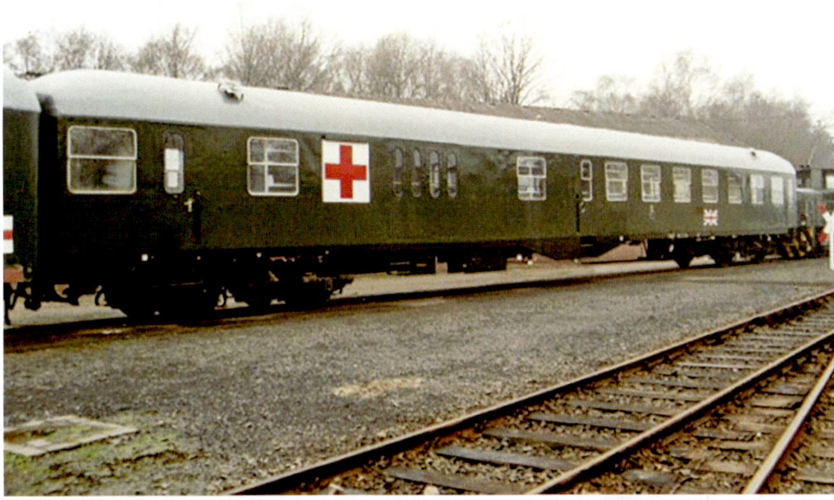

The prototype *Bcyl (Laz)* ward coach at 79 Railway Squadron RCT in 1990.

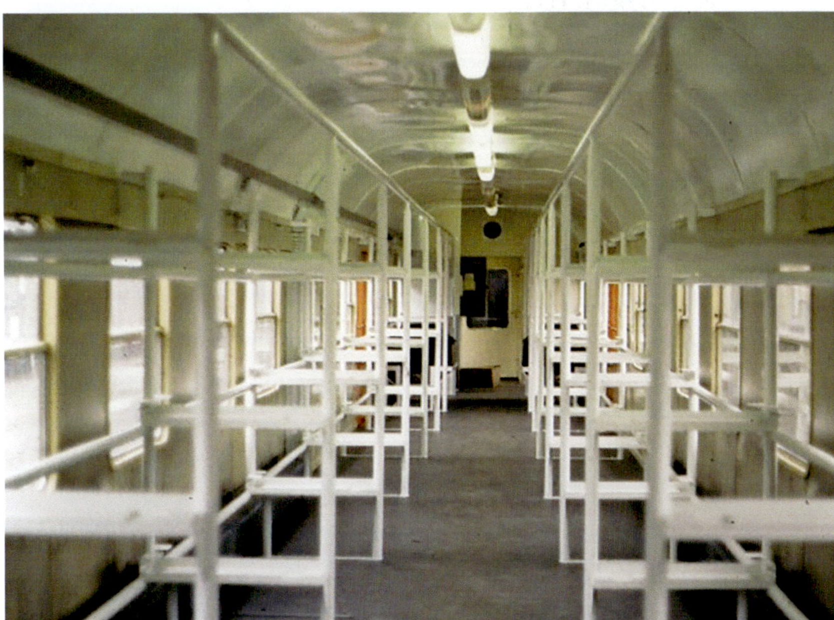

Stretcher frames to take forty stretchers within a *Bcyl (Laz)* ward coach.

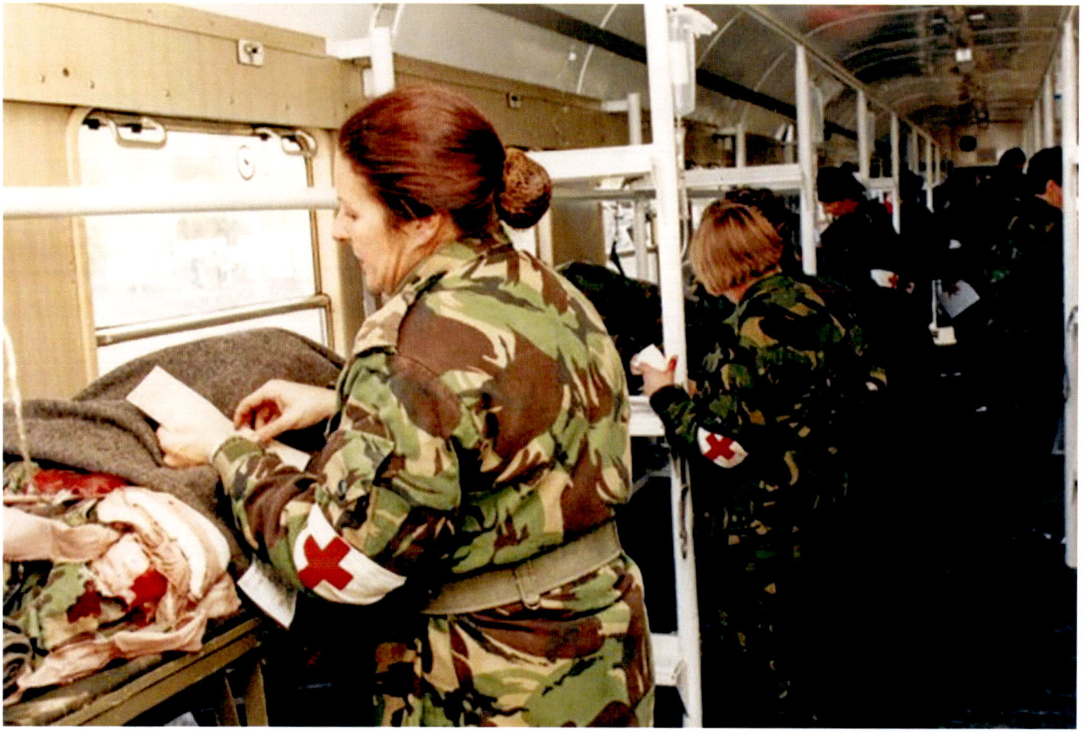

Nursing care within a *Bcyl (Laz)* ward coach on Exercise FLYING SCOT 93. (© Crown copyright)

Following their conversion this rolling stock fleet entered service with a new DB rolling stock designation of *Bcyl (Laz)*. These coaches had wide loading doors along with two water carriage packs per coach. The true operational water requirement of an ambulance train had been seriously underestimated for some years and this conversion rectified this shortcoming. These coaches proved to be an excellent conversion that provided a good patient ride, were very good for the staff to work on and would have given many more years of service had not the decision to disband all ambulance train capability intervened.

OTHER ROLLING STOCK REQUIREMENTS

In addition to the ambulance ward coaches, several other types of rolling stock were essential to complete ambulance train formations. These included kitchen diners, luggage vans and couchette coaches, the latter being required for both staff accommodation and walking casualties.

The British Army owned three kitchen diners which carried the DB rolling stock designation of *Wrüm*. They were not primarily allocated to ambulance train operations as they were committed to other military rail activity on mobilisation. However, when available these kitchen diners were utilised on ambulance train exercises. Usually painted in the British Army deep bronze-green, one of the three kitchen diners was upgraded internally in 1993 and repainted in RLC colours primarily for another military rail requirement. It was used in an ambulance train formation on Exercise FLYING SCOT 93 that visited Sennelager, Gutersloh and Hohne. With the drawdown of British Forces in BAOR this kitchen diner was disposed of and has been preserved and is operating on a German heritage railway.

Two utility coaches came to the British Army from the USATC in 1987. These provided heating and power to a train and were, on a few occasions, used in ambulance train formations although their primary commitment was to another British Army railway task so they would not be available for ambulance trains on mobilisation.

Every ambulance train also required a luggage van which had the generic DB rolling stock designation *Dm* and came in many variants. They were hired from the DB and depending on availability several different types including postal variants were used over the years. The role of these vans was to house the train command post along with bulk medical and general stores.

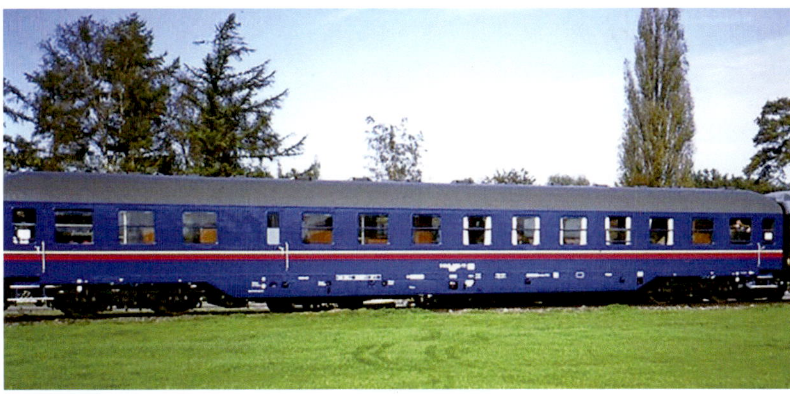

Kitchen diner at RAF Gutersloh during Exercise FLYING SCOT 93.

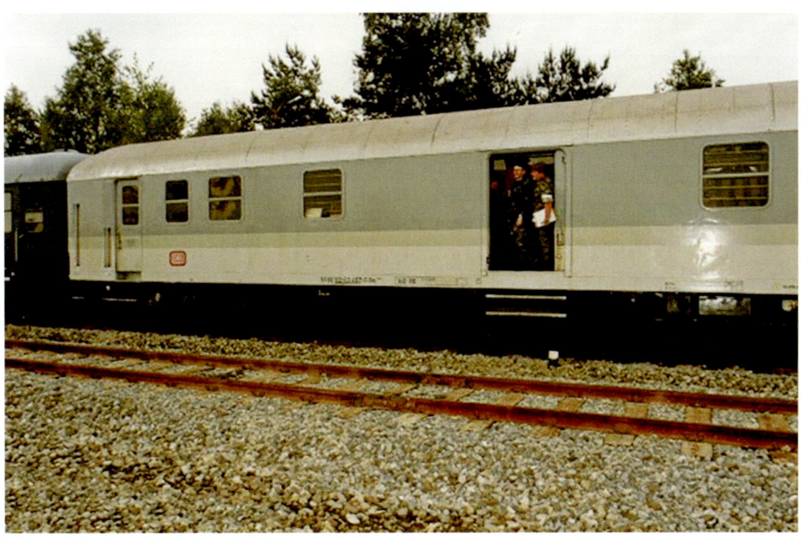

A hired DB luggage van in an ambulance train formation in the Arsbeck Training Area.

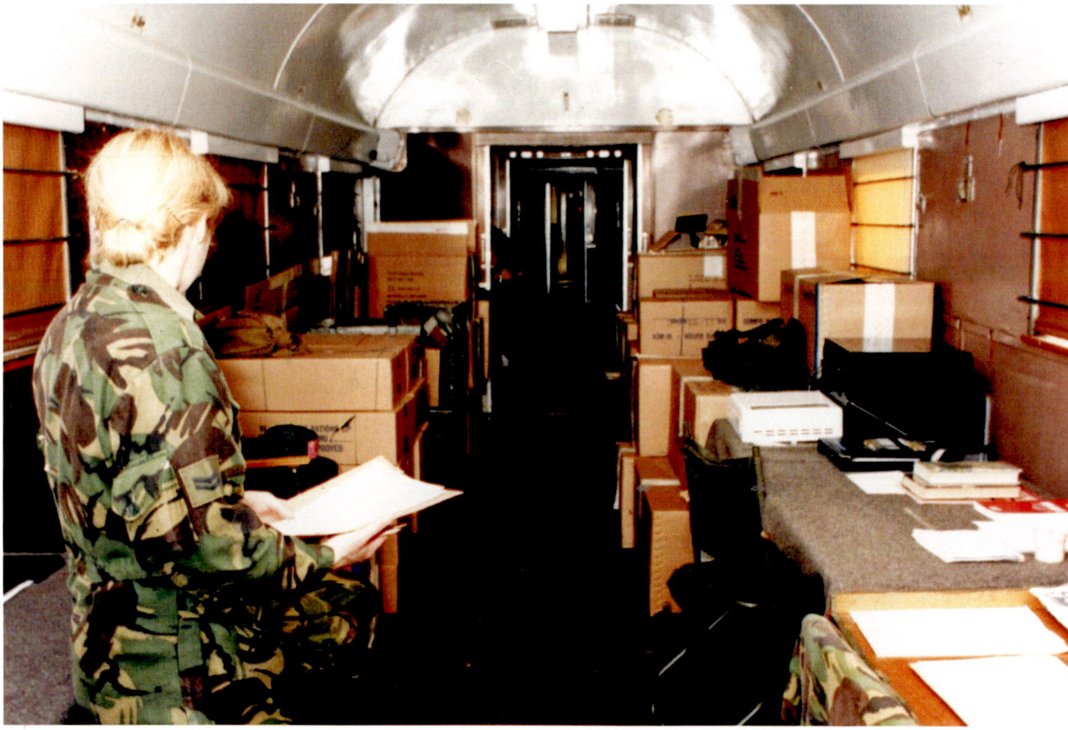

Train Command Post within a DB luggage van with stores beyond. (© Crown copyright)

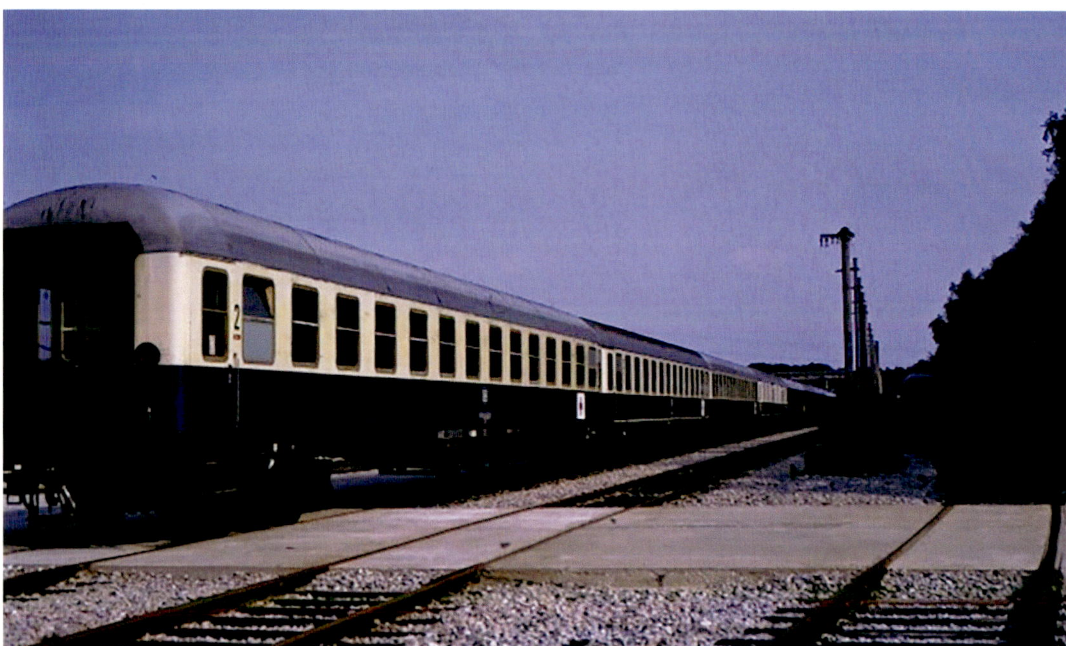

Hired DB couchette coaches used for staff accommodation and sitting casualties at 79 Railway Squadron RCT.

Couchette coaches were another essential part of an ambulance train formation. Also hired from the DB, they were used for both staff accommodation and walking casualties. When used in an ambulance train formation Red Cross emblems were hung where destinations panels would normally have been displayed on the outside of each coach. The thinking behind the use of couchette coaches rather than sitting stock for the walking casualties was that considering the potential length of journeys all casualties should be allowed to lie down.

HOME AMBULANCE TRAINS

In the days of the Cold War there was a well-defined Joint Theatre Plan, JTP 201, for the return of casualties in the event of hostilities. This plan would utilise road ambulances and coaches along with the BAOR ambulance trains, cross-Channel ferry assets taken up from trade and ambulance trains within the UK in order to distribute casualties around the country. There was, however, no dedicated ambulance train rolling stock available during the Cold War and reliance was placed on the transition to war (TTW) period to allow conversion of stock. Although the number of types and trains required had been scoped in detail, conversion plans were far less firm.

In 1982 a trial took place to validate a potential conversion kit that could be readily manufactured during TTW to convert the required number of carriages. British Rail engineers designed a conversion to fit an FO Mk 2f coach and a trial rake of stock was delivered to Ludgershall Military Sidings, in Wiltshire, on 18 October 1982. The conversion was designed to take twenty-four stretchers per coach.

It had long been known that no stretcher would fit through the doors of BR passenger rolling stock of the time and a newspaper van with the rolling stock designation of NLX was part of the rake to allow the double-door access that was necessary to load stretchers onto the train. Once in the van, a stretcher would need to be carried along the train to an appropriate berth.

Ambulance Train Squadron personnel only ever undertook static trials of the conversion in October 1984 at Ludgershall Military Sidings along with participation in two medical formation exercises. These were Exercise TARTAN OCTOPUS 87 and TARTAN OCTOPUS 88, where the conversion was again used in a static role at Stirling Station in Scotland.

It was subsequently planned that this conversion would form the basis for the home ambulance trains required under JTP 201. However, as far as is known, no stockpile of conversion kits was ever built and it was not long before the newspaper industry stopped using rail for their distribution. The NLX and other similar vans were withdrawn, and the Mk 2 passenger stock was gradually replaced by newer models. Sadly, the single prototype conversion kit that had been trialled disappeared without trace, although a technical record survived.[5]

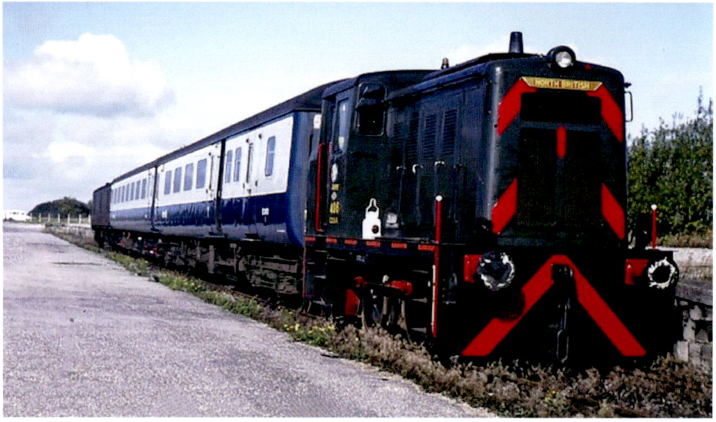

Trial rake of proposed home ambulance train rolling stock at Ludgershall Military Sidings behind Army locomotive 406 on 18 October 1982.

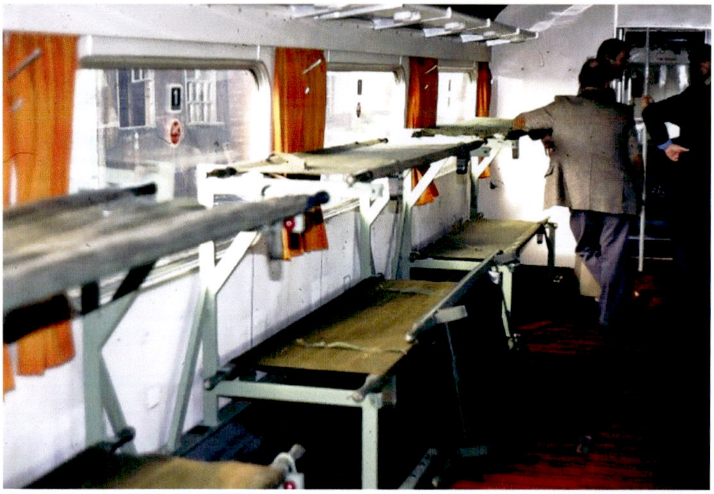

Prototype stretcher conversion of an FO Mk 2f coach designed to take twenty-four stretchers.

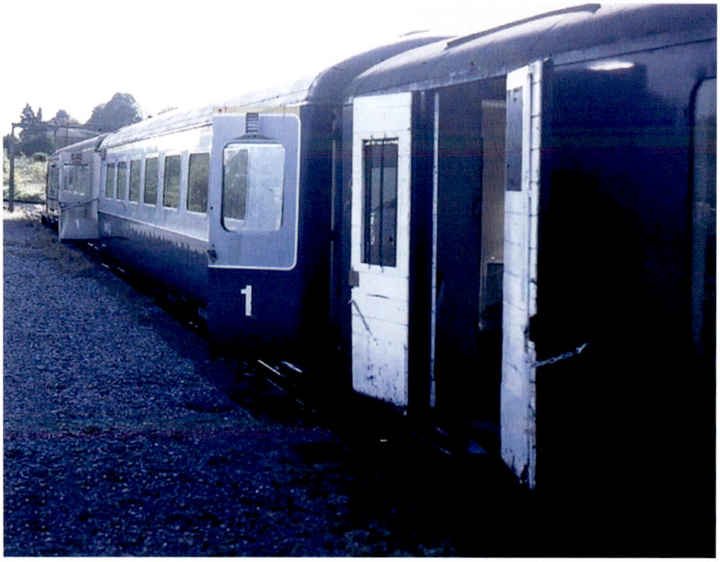

The NLX newspaper sorting van showing the double-door access needed to load stretchers.

8
The Future

This history of the use of ambulance trains by British Forces had a natural end point in 1995 when all British Army ambulance train capability was disbanded at the end of the Cold War. At the time of disbandment a senior British Army commander told the author that: 'We shall never need ambulance trains again'. History may well prove that individual wrong.

Mention should be made of the Covid-19 pandemic, which began in 2019 and the WHO formally ended in May 2023.[1] Whilst cases and variants continue to circulate, and the end of any pandemic is never easy to define, as at August 2024, Covid-19 had caused over 7 million deaths worldwide and ranks as the fifth-deadliest pandemic in history. The value of rail to transport patients was rediscovered during the pandemic, first by France in 2020 when patients were moved, using SNCF TGV train sets, from areas of high case numbers to areas of the country that had available intensive care facilities.

There is active talk once again about the needs for ambulance train capabilities, both military and civilian, throughout Europe. The invasion of Ukraine by Russia in 2022 has led to fears of a wider conflict in Europe and with the increasing instability in the Middle East, even talk of a Third World War.

Russia invaded Ukraine on 24 February 2022 and despite damage to rolling stock, infrastructure and loss of life, the state-owned Ukrainian Railways continues to deliver a service in the same way many railway companies have throughout previous wars. Ukrainian Railways have a mixture of broad- and standard-gauge networks and have to date evacuated over 2 million people displaced by the war.[2]

In late 2023 Ukrainian Railways constructed an autonomous Food Train with philanthropic funds from overseas. It has the capability of delivering 10,000 hot meals per day in regions that have suffered power outages and infrastructure damage. This six-coach train feeds residents as well as emergency service workers and can work autonomously for up to seven days.[3] Whilst this will have been seen by some as new and innovative, history tells us about the *Labetrains* used during the First World War by the Austro-Hungarian Empire. These were mobile feeding trains of which twenty-five were in operation by May 1916 and were located at strategic points around the rail network specifically to service hospital and ambulance trains.[4] Without doubt what Ukrainian Railways have done is an important concept for other agencies to develop in the future in order to support refugees and displaced persons and yet again shows the potential of rail.

Ukrainian Railways have also provided rolling stock for the evacuation of casualties, as did Poland. As is so often the case, the early efforts were improvised with little or no formal conversion of rolling stock. The use of rail commenced in March 2022 with a minimally adapted train operated by *Médecins Sans Frontières* (MSF), an independent humanitarian non-governmental organisation that was already working in Ukraine. During 2023 MSF and Ukrainian Railways produced an eight-coach MEDEVAC train that was fully converted for role. All the required elements such as power, water and oxygen supplies were addressed and patient care capability up to intensive care level provided.[5]

There is indeed a future for casualty evacuation by rail, but it needs to embrace both modern railway technology and also the modern demands of medicine of all specialities. Whilst trauma will be at the forefront of people's minds, in the conflict situation it is important to remember that the full range of medical conditions will be seen in displaced populations. There has to also be an acceptance that the use of rail cannot really be achieved on an ad hoc basis, but detailed planning and conversion of rolling stock is essential for its effective use and this takes time.

From the medical standpoint medical evacuation by rail needs to encompass all classes of patients and future trains should be of modular design and construction to allow flexibility. Four categories of patients should be planned for. Firstly, the walking patients or those in wheelchairs who can sit throughout their journey and who will require low levels of medical and nursing care. They will require adequate sitting space and leg room along with safe fixings for wheelchairs. Secondly there will be the stretcher patients where the capacity will be dictated by the conversion frames into which stretchers may be fixed. The third and fourth categories are the high dependency and intensive care patients. These both require adjustable-height patient trolleys with space to work around the patient along with increasing levels of technical equipment and staff to patient ratios. The ability to manage both pre- and post-operative ventilated patients will form the basis of any intensive care capability. The much-improved ride characteristics of modern generations of railway rolling stock will also significantly enhance patient care.

EPILOGUE

In addition to where there has been detailed history this book has attempted to pull together many of those one or two sentence references to the use of ambulance trains in various campaigns and show that they were part of a much bigger and organised whole. It is sad that so much detail of the use of rail has been lost in the mists of time. This book also aims to recognise, with gratitude, the dedication and service of the staff of all those trains wherever they served.

This history has shown how well ambulance trains have served earlier generations and there is no doubt they could do so again in the future. There was a much-quoted mantra during the Cold War that 'ambulance trains do not move anyone, anywhere fast but they move large numbers long distances in warmth, light and receiving medical and nursing care'. The same will be true of future generations of ambulance trains, but with far greater emphasis on enhanced levels of clinical care for the right patient and delivering them to the right destination.

Notes

PREFACE

1. Bricknell, Martin and Vassallo, David, *Researching Modern Military History* in *Topics in the History of Medicine*, 3 (2023), pp. 278–95.

EARLY DAYS OF THE USE OF RAILWAYS

1. Cooke, Brian, *The Grand Crimean Central Railway*, 2nd edn (Knutsford: Cavalier House, 1997).
2. *Ibid.*, p. 73.
3. Puzzilla, Anthony, *Hospital Trains and Vessels during the Civil War* (Manchester: Canoe Tree Press, 2020), p. 121.
4. Austin, David, *Ambulance Trains in War* in *Southern Way*, 42 (Crecy Publishing, 2018), pp. 42–57.
5. Plumridge, John, *Hospital Ships and Ambulance Trains* (London: Seeley Service and Co., 1975), p. 90.
6. Pratt, Edwin A., *The Rise of Rail Power in War and Conquest* (London: P. S. King and Son, 1915), p. 95.
7. *Journal of the Statistical Society of London*, 38 (June 1875), pp. 249–52.
8. *British Medical Journal*, 2, 822 (30 September 1876), p. 440.
9. Marden, Dave, *The Hidden Railways of Portsmouth and Gosport* (Southampton: Kestrel Railway Books, 2014).
10. Maurice, J. F., *The Campaign of 1882 in Egypt*. Facsimile reproduction by Naval & Military Press of an original published in 1887, p. 5.
11. Rainbow, J. Julian, *British Military Railways in the Egyptian Campaign of 1882*. Unpublished.
12. War Office, *Manual for the Medical Staff Corps* (London: HMSO, 1894), p. 141.
13. War Office, *Royal Army Medical Corps Training* (London: HMSO, 1908), p. 38.

SOUTH AFRICAN WAR

1. Melville, C., *Continental requirements for the transportation of sick and wounded by rail. Royal United Services Institution Journal* (1898), 42, pp. 560–94.

2. De Villiers, J. C., *Healers, Helpers and Hospitals: A History of Military Medicine in the Anglo-Boer War* (Pretoria: Protea Book House, 2008), p. 311.
3. *Ibid.*, pp. 329–30.
4. *Report by the Central British Red Cross Committee on Voluntary Organisations in aid of the sick and wounded during the South African War* (London: HMSO, 1902), p. 32.
5. Hypher, J., Wheeler, C., and Wheeler, S., *Birmingham Railway Carriage and Wagon Company* (Runpast Publishing, 1995), p. 9.
6. Plumridge, John H., *Hospital Ships and Ambulance Trains* (London: Seeley Service, 1975), p. 173.
7. British Red Cross, *op. cit.*, p. 137.
8. Bonham-Carter, Gerald, British Red Cross Museum and Archives. Accession number: WAN/15/7/14 30 (December 1900).
9. British Red Cross, *op. cit.*, p. 139.
10. *St John in Focus* (London: Museum of the Order of St John, 1987), p. 15.
11. *Royal Commission on the Care and Treatment of the Sick and Wounded in the South African Campaign* (London: HMSO, 1901), p. 13.
12. Prime, Peter, *The History of the Medical and Hospital Services of the Anglo-Boer War 1899–1902* (Anglo-Boer War Philatelic Society, 1998), p. 176.
13. De Villiers, J. C., *op. cit.*, p. 375.
14. Prime, Peter, *op. cit.*, p. 69.
15. Fairman, John R., *Netley Hospital and its Railways* (Southampton: Kingfisher Railway Productions, 1984), p. 17.
16. Hoare, Philip, *Spike Island: The Memory of a Military Hospital* (London: Fourth Estate, 2002), p. 175.
17. Fairman, John R., *op. cit.*, p. 43.
18. 'Second Boer War', *Wikipedia* (accessed: 29 February 2024).
19. Royal Commission 1901, *op. cit.*, p. 16.
20. *British Medical Journal*, 10 October 1903, pp. 930–34.

FIRST WORLD WAR

1. Luard, K. E, *Diary of A Nursing Sister on the Western Front 1914–1915* (Blackwood, 1915), p. 69.
2. Pratt, Edwin, A., *British Railways and the Great War. Organisation, Efforts, Difficulties and Achievements,* 1921, Volume 1 (facsimile reprint by Naval & Military Press Ltd), pp. 196–97.
3. Plumridge, John H., *Hospital Ships and Ambulance Trains* (London: Seeley Service, 1975) pp. 130–31.
4. Pratt, Edwin A., *op. cit.,* Volume 1, pp. 219–20.
5. *Ibid.*, p. 198.
6. *Ibid.*, p. 212.
7. *Ibid.*, pp. 213–14.

8. *Ibid.*, p. 221.
9. Plumridge, John, H., *op. cit.*, p. 131.
10. *Ibid.*, p. 128.
11. Pratt, Edwin A., *op. cit.,* Volume 1, p. 216.
12. Pratt, Edwin A., *op. cit.,* Volume 2, pp. 562–63.
13. Millard, P. A., *LNWR Great War Ambulance Trains*. Premium Portfolio No. 11, LNWR Society Publication (1993), p. 39.
14. Pratt, Edwin A., *op. cit.*, Volume 2, p. 571.
15. *Ibid.*, p. 566.
16. *Ibid.*, p. 563.
17. Plumridge, John, H., *op. cit.*, pp. 126–27.
18. Friel, Charles, *Personal communication*, October–December 2024.
19. *Reports by the Joint War Committee and the Joint War Finance Committee of the British Red Cross Society and the Order of St John of Jerusalem in England on Voluntary Aid rendered to the Sick and Wounded at Home and Abroad and to British Prisoners of War. 1914–1919* (London: HMSO, 1921) (facsimile reprint by Naval & Military Press Ltd), p. 189.
20. *Ibid.*, p. 191.
21. Moore, George A., *The Birth and Early Days of our Ambulance Trains in France, August 1914*, 2nd edn (London: John Bale, Sons and Danielsson Ltd, 1922).
22. *Ibid.*, p. 5.
23. *Ibid.*, p. 5.
24. *Ibid.*, p. 5.
25. Plumridge, John H., *op. cit.*, p. 175.
26. Pratt, Edwin A., *op. cit.*, Volume 1, p. 204.
27. Plumridge, John H., *op. cit.*, pp. 183–84.
28. *Ibid.*, pp. 175–76.
29. Geldard, David, 'First World War Ambulance Trains' in *Journal of the Transport Ticket Society*, 619, August 2015 (The Transport Ticket Society), pp. 315–22.
30. Waters, Paul E. and Rainbow, J. Julian (eds), *British Military Railways Overseas in the Great War* (Chippenham: Mainline and Maritime Ltd, 2018), pp. 325–26.
31. Pratt, Edwin A., *op. cit.*, Volume 1, p. 208.
32. Geldard, David, *op. cit.*, p. 315.
33. Plumridge, John H., *op. cit.*, p. 112.
34. Geldard, David, op. cit., p. 317.
35. Pratt, Edwin A., *op. cit.*, Volume 1, p. 210.
36. Hoggett, Kevin, *Rails across the Sea* (Chippenham: Mainline and Maritime Ltd, 2020), p. 11.
37. Pegler, Martin, *Soldiers' Songs and Slang of the Great War* (Oxford: Osprey Publishing, 2014), p. 38.
38. Muir, Ward, *Observations of an Orderly* (Liskeard: Diggory Press, 2006), p. 44.

39. Macpherson, W. G. and Mitchell, T. J., *History of the Great War based on Official Documents – Medical Services* (1923) (facsimile reproduction by Naval & Military Press Ltd), Volume 4, pp. 656–58.
40. High, Peter L. (ed.), *Hospital Barges in France – Correspondence from a Nursing Sister with the British Expeditionary Force during World War 1* (Perth: Chavril Press).
41. Higgins, Jeremy, *Casualty Evacuation for the Somme* (Warwick: Helion and Company, 2020), p. 176.
42. HRH The Duke of Windsor, *A King's Story* (Cassel and Co., 1951), pp. 118–19.
43. British Religious Society of Friends. Supplement to *The Friend* (1916), pp. i–xii.
44. *Ibid.*, p. iv.
45. Personnel of Ambulance Train 16, *A Train Errant being the Experiences of a Voluntary Unit in France and an Anthology from their Magazine* (Hertford: Simpson and Co. Ltd, 1919).
46. Friends' Ambulance Unit, No. 17 Ambulance Train, *Lines of Communication – A Souvenir Volume* (London: Wightman and Co. Ltd, 1919).
47. Personnel of Ambulance Train 16, *op. cit.*, p. 2.
48. *Ibid.*, p. 6.
49. *Ibid.*, p. 7.
50. Friends' Ambulance Unit, No. 17 Ambulance Train, *op. cit.*, p. 8.
51. *Ibid.*, p. 86.
52. Palfreeman, Linda, *Friends in Flanders* (Brighton: Sussex Academic Press, 2017), p. 179.
53. Pratt, Edwin A., *op. cit.*, Volume 1, p. 207.
54. Faulkner, J. N., and Williams, R. A., *The LSWR in the Twentieth Century* (Newton Abbott: David & Charles, 1988), p. 120.
55. Geldard, David, *op. cit.,* p. 321.
56. Macpherson, W. G., *op. cit.*, Volume 1, p. 281.
57. *Ibid.*, p. 282.
58. *Ibid.*, p. 299.
59. *Ibid.*, p. 303.
60. Pratt, Edwin A., *op. cit.*, Volume 1, p. 79.
61. *Ibid.*, p. 80.
62. *Ibid.*, pp. 134–35.
63. *Ibid.*, p. 150.
64. *Ibid.*, p. 155.
65. *Ibid.*, pp. 156–57.
66. Waters, Paul E. and Rainbow, J. Julian (eds), *op. cit.*, p. 323.
67. *Ibid.*, p. 323.
68. *Ibid.*, p. 69.
69. Civil, Alan and Etherington, Roy, *The Railway Products of Baguley-Drewry Ltd and its Predecessors* (Industrial Railway Society, 2008), pp. 57–58.
70. *The Railway Gazette*, 21 September 1920, pp. 101–07.
71. Macpherson, W. G., *op. cit.*, Volume 2, pp. 329–30.

72. *Ibid.*, p. 359.
73. *Ibid.*, p. 359.
74. 'Sinai and Palestine Campaign', *Wikipedia* (accessed: 13 November 2024).
75. Macpherson, W. G., *op. cit.*, Volume 2, pp. 433–34.
76. *Ibid.*, p. 420.
77. *Ibid.*, pp. 427–28.
78. *Ibid.*, p. 457.
79. Rainbow, Julian, 'The Evacuation of the Sick and Wounded on the Palestine Lines of Communications' in *The British Overseas Railways Journal,* 44 (Summer 2020), pp. 124–33.
80. Macpherson, W. G., *op. cit.,* Volume 4, p. 420.
81. *Ibid.*, p. 476.
82. *Ibid.*, p. 531.
83. *Ibid.*, p. 543.
84. www.thirdsector.co.uk/1914-1918-charities-help-in-ww1 (accessed: 12 February 2024).
85. www.em.wikipedia.org/wiki/Australian_Comforts_Fund (accessed: 17 March 2024).

SECOND WORLD WAR

1. Plumridge, John H., *Hospital Ships and Ambulance Trains* (London: Seeley Service, 1975), p. 138.
2. Dunn, C. L., *History of the Second World War, United Kingdom Medical Series. The Emergency Medical Services, 1951* (facsimile reprint by Naval & Military Press Ltd).
3. Hudson, Leonard, Personal communications, 1992.
4. Plumridge, John H., *op. cit.*, p. 139.
5. Bell, R., *History of British Railways during the War 1939–45* (*The Railway Gazette*, 1946), p. 196.
6. Darwin, Bernard, *War on the Line*, 1946 (reprinted Middleton Press, 1984), p. 150.
7. Dunn, C. L., *op. cit.*, Volume 1, p. 279.
8. *Ibid.*, p. 289.
9. Holt, F. Trevor, Personal communication, 1995.
10. Dunn, C. L., *op. cit.*, Volume 1, p. 85.
11. Moon, George, 'Ex-LSWR Ambulance Cars in WD Service' in *Military Railway Study Group Bulletin* 34, (Nov/Dec 2024), pp. 152–53.
12. Bayliff, Rob J. E., Personal communication, January 2025.
13. Friel, Charles, Personal communication, January 2025.
14. *The Railway Gazette*, 10 November 1939, p. 608.
15. Crew, F. A., *History of the Second World War, United Kingdom Medical Services. The Army Medical Services Campaigns, 1953* (facsimile reprint by Naval & Military Press Ltd), Volume 1, p. 9.

16. *Ibid.*, p. 15.
17. *Ibid.*, p. 24.
18. Maginniss, Clem, *A Great Feat of Improvisation* (Warwick: Helion and Co. Ltd, 2021), p. 347.
19. Alves, William T., *Supporting the British Expeditionary Force: The Royal Engineer Units in France 1939–1940* (Donington: Shaun Tynas, 2012), p. 15.
20. Crew, F. A., *op. cit.*, Volume 1, p. 25.
21. *Ibid.*, p. 45.
22. McBryde, Brenda, *Quiet Heroines* (Saffron Walden: Cakebread Publications, 1989), p. 20.
23. LMS Carriage and Wagon Office, Wolverton, Document detailing rolling stock used in overseas ambulance trains, dated 1 March 1944 updated after Dunkirk (in author's archive).
24. 'Dunkirk Evacuation', *Wikipedia* (accessed: 27 September 2024).
25. Dunn, C. L., *op. cit.*, Volume 1, p. 100.
26. Maginniss, Clem, *op. cit.*, p. 510.
27. 'Landing Ship Tank', *Wikipedia* (accessed: 8 December 2024).
28. Dunn, C. L., *op. cit.*, Volume 1, pp. 163–65.
29. *Ibid.*, p. 290.
30. Mitchell, Vic, *Railways to Victory* (Midhurst: Middleton Press,1998), p. 76.
31. Whitelock, A., *Personal communication*, 1992.
32. Shrivenham Heritage Society, shrivenhamheritagesociety.co.uk (accessed: 23 December 2024).
33. Crew, F. A., *op. cit.*, Volume 1, p. 407.
34. *Ibid.*, p. 416–17.
35. *Ibid.*, p. 479.
36. *Ibid.*, p. 464.
37. Crew, F. A., *op. cit.*, Volume 2, p. 269.
38. *Ibid.*, p. 287.
39. Lloyd Williamson, J., 'Ambulance Trains in Algeria and Tunisia' in *Railway Magazine*, 90, (Jan/Feb 1944), pp. 3–6.
40. Crew, F. A., *op. cit.*, Volume 2, p. 308.
41. Lloyd Williamson, J., *op. cit.*, p. 6.
42. Crew, F. A., *op. cit.*, Volume 2, p. 313.
43. 'Italian Campaign (WW2)', *Wikipedia* (accessed: 4 October 2024).
44. Crew, F. A., *op. cit.*, Volume 3, p. 101.
45. *Ibid.*, p. 172.
46. *Ibid.*, p. 181.
47. *Ibid.*, p. 219.
48. Crew, F. A., *op. cit.*, Volume 1, p. 489.
49. Plumridge, John H., *op. cit.*, p. 143.
50. Crew, F. A., *op. cit.*, Volume 5, pp. 11, 32, 71, 586, 587, 595.
51. *Ibid.*, p. 8.
52. *Ibid.*, p. 11.

53. *Ibid.*, p. 42.
54. *Ibid.*, p. 87.

POST-SECOND WORLD WAR

1. Fairman, John R., *Netley Hospital and its Railways* (Southampton: Kingfisher Railway Productions, 1984), p. 70.

KOREAN WAR

1. Taylor, Karen, *8138th Army Unit Hospital Trains* (Lacey: Boot Top Books, 2021), p. 3.
2. Sibul, Eric, 'Medical Railroading during the Korean War 1950–1953' in *Railroad History*, 204 (Spring-Summer 2001), p. 54.
3. Taylor, Karen, *op. cit.,* pp. 48–64.
4. O'Brien, David, Personal communication (October 1988).
5. McNair, Jilly, *A British Army Nurse in the Korean War* (Stroud: Tempus Publishing, 2007), p. 142.
6. 'Korean War', *Wikipedia* (accessed: 11 September 2021).

COLD WAR

1. 'NATO', *Wikipedia* (accessed: 18 August 2024).
2. Chrystal, Paul, *British Army of the Rhine, The BAOR 1945–1993* (Barnsley: Pen & Sword Military, 2018).
3. Johnston, Peter, *British Forces in Germany the lived experience* (London: Profile Books Ltd, 2019).
4. Watson, Graham E., and Rinaldi, Richard A., *The British Army in Germany (BAOR and after): An Organisational History 1947–2004* (Tiger Lily Publications LLC, 2005).
5. British Rail, *Instructions for the fitting of stretcher frames*. Undated (in author's archive).

THE FUTURE

1. 'Covid-19 Pandemic', *Wikipedia* (accessed: 9 August 2024).
2. 'Ukrainian Railways', *Wikipedia* (accessed: 9 August 2024).
3. 'Ukrainian Railways', *Wikipedia* (accessed: 9 August 2024).
4. '*Ein mobile Labetrain*', *Die Zeit*, 20 July 1915.
5. Walvrens, S., Zharkova, A., *et al., Characteristics of Medical Evacuation by Train in Ukraine, 2022. JAMA* Network Open. 2023: 6 (6): e2319726.